# Stressed Out

## About Pharmacology

### Richard Freedberg, RN, MSN, MPA

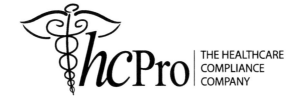

THE HEALTHCARE
COMPLIANCE
COMPANY

*Stressed Out About Pharmacology* is published by HCPro, Inc.

Copyright ©2008 HCPro, Inc.

All rights reserved. Printed in the United States of America.     5   4   3   2   1

ISBN: 978-1-60146-121-6

HCPro, Inc., provides information resources for the healthcare industry.

HCPro, Inc., is not affiliated in any way with The Joint Commission, which owns the JCAHO and Joint Commission trademarks.

Richard Freedberg, RN, MSN, MPA, Author
Ken Rohde, Contributing Author
Michael Briddon, Editor
Jamie Gisonde, Executive Editor
Emily Sheahan, Group Publisher
Shane Katz, Cover Designer
Mike Mirabello, Senior Graphic Artist
David Clemente, Layout Artist
Audrey Doyle, Copyeditor
Liza Banks, Proofreader
Darren Kelly, Books Production Supervisor
Susan Darbyshire, Art Director
Claire Cloutier, Production Manager
Jean St. Pierre, Director of Operations

Advice given is general. Readers should consult professional counsel for specific legal, ethical, or clinical questions. Arrangements can be made for quantity discounts. For more information, contact:

HCPro, Inc.
P.O. Box 1168
Marblehead, MA 01945
Telephone: 800/650-6787 or 781/639-1872
Fax: 781/639-2982
E-mail: *customerservice@hcpro.com*

**Visit Stressed Out Nurses: *www.StressedOutNurses.com***

02/2008
21388

# Dedication

To **Sally**

# Acknowledgments

The author wishes to acknowledge the attentive guidance and inexhaustibly good-natured support from Michael Briddon, managing editor at HCPro, Inc.

# Contents

# Contents

# How to use this book

What if there was a book that explained complex nursing topics in an easy-to-understand manner and in an accessible format? That's the premise behind the *Stressed Out…*series. Solid references with a bit of a sense of humor and the understanding that a lighthearted approach to learning makes the whole thing more enjoyable.

To help you navigate through the book, you will find the following icons highlighting a particular passage:

 **Don't forget:** A little reminder about something of importance.

 **Don't panic:** Take a deep breath and relax. Get ready for a little reassurance.

 **Tip:** A bit of inside information, a hint, or helpful advice.

 **Watch out:** Word to the wise; this is a warning.

 **Click:** This icon refers you to a helpful Web site, where you may find further information on the topic.

 **Did you know:** An interesting fact that helps to add some perspective.

**Happy Nursing! Now you're ready to get started.**

# About the author

## Richard Freedberg, RN, MSN, MPA

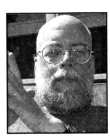 **Richard Freedberg, RN, MSN, MPA,** has earned an associate's degree in nursing from Lansing Community College, a bachelor of science in zoology from Michigan State University, a bachelor of science in nursing from the University of Detroit-Mercy, a master of science in nursing from Eastern Michigan University, a master of public administration from Western Michigan University, and is a doctoral student in interdisciplinary health studies at Western Michigan University.

His clinical experience includes staff nursing and management roles in medical-surgical and mental health acute-care settings, home-care nursing, and medical intermediate care. He is currently professor of mental health nursing at Lansing Community College in Lansing, MI. In addition, he continues to practice in a clinical setting (nursing is a stunningly incredible way to spend your life!).

*Author photo by Sean Freedberg*

## About the contributor

**Kenneth R. Rohde** is a senior consultant for The Greeley Company, a division of HCPro, Inc. He brings more than 27 years of experience in quality management to his work with hospitals and medical centers across the country.

Mr. Rohde's roles in performance improvement and project management make him uniquely qualified to assist medical staffs and hospital leaders in developing solutions to their toughest challenges. He instructs, speaks, and consults in the areas of error reduction strategies, root cause analysis, improving performance through process simplification, error reduction through effective procedure writing, apparent cause analysis, engineering effectiveness and error reduction, failure modes and effects analysis, effective data collection, analysis and trending, patient safety evaluation and improvement, change management, corrective action program evaluation and redesign, human performance evaluations, and procedure error reduction. Mr. Rohde also specializes in technology-based approaches to preventing human errors and analyzing performance data.

Mr. Rohde holds a B.S. in mechanical engineering from the University of Hawaii.

## About the reviewer

**Jason Corcoran, PharmD, BCPS,** is the clinical pharmacy specialist for the Inova Fairfax Hospital for Children in Falls Church, VA. He has more than 10 years of pharmacy work experience, including the past five years in practice as a pediatric pharmacist.

Dr. Corcoran began his career as a pharmacy technician in his hometown of Richmond, VA, and an interest in the unique aspects of providing medications to children led him to pursue post-graduate residency training. After completing hospital pharmacy practice and pediatric specialty residencies at The Johns Hopkins Hospital in 2003, he was a clinical pharmacy specialist in the pediatric intensive care unit at the Children's Hospital, Cleveland Clinic.

Dr. Corcoran received his doctor of pharmacy degree from Virginia Commonwealth University in 2001. He is a member of several pharmaceutical organizations including the American Society of Health-System Pharmacists, the American College of Clinical Pharmacy, and the Pediatric Pharmacy Advocacy Group.

# Introduction

## Welcome, class. Please be seated . . .

Let's just put it out there at the beginning: Pharmacology class never ends. Suddenly in need of some good news? Okay, here you go: This will be the best and most fun pharmacology course you will ever take!

Greetings!

What follows is a brief introduction outlining the task we are about to undertake. Most likely, you are taking pharmacology—concurrently with your nursing courses—as a pre-nursing or nursing student. Or, you have just begun your nursing career and are assailed by those doubts we all have experienced: "I really don't know enough to be a nurse and sooner or later 'they' will find out!"

It is completely natural to be anxious. Remember though, a little anxiety is good because it increases our attentiveness and processing ability. Pharmacology is a challenging subject, and there is a ton to learn and remember, but let's reframe how we look at this situation: Instead of seeing pharmacology only as a required class that happens to us and as something out of our control, let's view it as it really is—an intriguing and exciting area of study that thousands of students and future nurses become familiar with each year. And guess what? You can be successful, too!

One of the very cool things about being a nurse is that our practice changes and evolves as new treatments are introduced. In these days of rapid information dissemination thanks to the Internet, we work on the cutting edge. "Wait a minute," you say, "does that mean I am stuck studying pharmacology forever?" "YES, isn't that AWESOME!" (Sorry for shouting.)

Pharmacology class never ends, but you will never be expected to know everything because it is always changing. Accept and take comfort in that! *Stressed Out About Pharmacology* will show you what kinds of things you need to know and how you can learn them and will help prepare you to confidently maintain pharmacological competency for the rest of your nursing career.

It's time to begin our class . . .

# Part One

This interacts with this, and that interacts with that. Make sure to do this. Don't forget about that. It's no secret that pharmacology can create instant stress and headaches. This section will lay out the basics and provide some creative techniques to help you master all these concepts.

# Chapter 1

# There is just too much stuff for my brain!

Have you ever thought that about pharmacology? That there is just too much stuff to know? Too much stuff to learn?

First, there is the language. By now, you have perused your pharmacology text. You've heard of pharmacokinetics, loop diuretics, mood stabilizing agents, beta 2 adrenergic antagonists, etc. Did you get the impression you were reading a foreign language? Well, you were. It's true! Now, let's look at that for a minute. The language is indeed different and complex, but it is predictable, precise, and accessible. Each of the words or terms used above has a unique and dependable interpretation. You will understand it with a smidge of preparation.

**Don't panic:** There is a way to learn all this information.

Instead of trying to take in an entire section or chapter and letting the mass of new words give you anxiety and frustration, sort them and take each one by one. Learn each new term as you go, and put it into context to help you remember. For example, learn

- Receptor types as a group

- Drugs by class

- Drugs within a class by prototype

- Side effects by body system or receptor type, and so on

**Tip:** Flash cards are not just for third grade. When you run into a new term or drug, make a flash card. Carry them with you. Go through them whenever you get a chance. And remember to shuffle them often so you learn the content and not just the order!

## A drug by any other name . . .

P-isobutylhydratropic acid, ibuprofen, Motrin®, Advil®, Amersol®, and Nuprin® all refer to the same substance. What's up with that? We will look at drug names more closely in an upcoming lesson, but it is true that every drug has at least three names—and often more! Learning all of these can seem impossible, but don't despair—just keep a couple of things in mind.

First, in this class of ours, we will always sort drugs by generic and selected common trade names. Selected common trade names will be covered for each generic drug, but the brand names are of secondary importance. This is the best and easiest method to learn what we need to know to safely administer medications and to instruct our patients. This is an important lesson.

**Watch out:** Despite the temptation to learn only the brand names of commonly marketed drugs, it is crucial to learn the generic names to help ensure safe nursing practice.

Though pharmaceutical companies intentionally try to avoid it, some trade names are similar or sound as if they belong in another class of drugs. For example, Lasix® is a loop diuretic designed to help the kidneys get rid of extra fluid in the body, but Lexxel® is a combination drug used to treat hypertension (high blood pressure). We might confuse these brand names but would probably be better served if we learned the generics: furosemide (Lasix®) and enalapril/felodipine (Lexxel®).

Other confusing brand name examples are:

- Soma® (a muscle relaxant) competing in our memory with Sonata® (sleep aid)

- Celexa® (antidepressant) potentially confused with Celebrex® (nonsteroidal anti-inflammatory drug for arthritis)

Secondly, you clearly can't, and absolutely don't need to, know every drug name. But it is important to know how drugs are sorted and clustered. You will begin to build your basic familiarity with the drug groups or classes as we continue through future lessons. That is a most important first step. As we go, you will find that generic names within a drug class—particularly, the endings of names—often are similar enough to ease the learning process. You will see that you can learn the medication classes and the key prototype drugs that exemplify each class.

**Don't panic:** You will never be able to learn all of the drugs and no one expects you to! Not even a pharmacist can remember every drug name—take comfort in that!

## Is there as much material as I think?

The United States National Library of Medicine DailyMed Web site provides up-to-the-minute information on marketed drugs. Currently, the Web site contains information on 3,408 medications (as I type, but it changes minute to minute).

**Click:** Check the United States National Library of Medicine DailyMed Web site out for yourself. Enter a couple drug names at *http://dailymed.nlm.nih.gov.* Start with Adderall® and make your way to Zoloft®.

A typical comprehensive drug reference guidebook for nurses meant for daily use in clinical settings may well contain 1,500–2,000 pages. Epocrates Rx®, a medication reference and prescribing software program, uses twice the amount of space on the author's PDA than complete copies of the Bible, Henry David Thoreau's *Walden*, Lao-Tse's *Tao Te Ching*, and Walt Whitman's *Leaves of Grass* combined (yes, there are some books you should always carry with you)!

There truly is a huge amount of information, but it is all very well organized for easy use by the educated professional you will become. We are going to lay out a framework to simplify the classification of the large amount of drug information that the previous paragraphs alluded to. Again, medications are sometimes organized by class or use.

For example, in the cardiovascular category, there are groups of drugs that have different effects on the cardiovascular system. Antiarrhythmics affect the electrical part of the heart, while antihypertensives affect the blood pressure.

Groups of drugs that affect a body system in a certain way can be further broken down into drug classes based on their mechanism of action. For example, beta-blockers, calcium channel blockers, and angiotensin converting enzyme inhibitors are different classes of drugs that have an antihyperstensive effect on the cardiovascular system. Finally, within each drug class, there can be several drugs that have the same mechanism of action, but very different dosages, side effects, and therapeutic effectiveness.

Together, we will organize our drugs according to these body systems and use these categories:

- Neurological

- Mental health

- Cardiovascular

- Respiratory

- Gastrointestinal

- Urological

- Hormonal and reproductive

- Antimicrobials

- Antineoplastic (cancer)

- Anti-inflammatory and immunological

- Nutrition

Though drugs in each of these groups affect multiple systems, these familiar clusters will ease your studying.

As you begin your nursing career and then perhaps opt to specialize in a particular area—such as cardiac care or maternal-child health—it will be readily apparent that only certain medications are commonly used. Eventually, you will know them backwards, forwards, and inside out. You will find that information regarding less frequently employed drugs is effortlessly obtainable, and you will easily keep up with the newly approved drugs marketed each year. Be confident! All this is based on the assumption, however, that some careful preparation and diligent effort now will prepare you for that day.

How about a little math to get the ball rolling? No groaning back there!

# References

Aschenbrenner, D. and Venable, S. (2006). *Drug therapy in nursing.* Philadelphia: Lipponcott, Williams & Wilkins.

"Epocrates RX Pro." Drug Reference Guide for the PDA. Available at *www.epocrates.com/products/rxpro.* Accessed October 21, 2007.

U.S. National Library of Medicine, National Institutes of Health, U.S. Department of Health and Human Services. Available at *http://dailymed.nlm. nih.gov.* Accessed October 21, 2007.

# Chapter 2

# My, oh, my—it's math time!

Picture this scenario: A nursing student taking pharmacology is examining the upper respiratory medications chapter and notes that the usual dose of a common drug, Robitussin DM®, is 10 mL every four hours not to exceed 60 mL per day because of the risk of a serious potential adverse reaction called serotonin syndrome. She carefully memorizes this but wonders exactly what 10 mL is in terms of household measures. (She knows that none of her future patients are likely to know it either!)

And then imagine this one: The diligent pharmacology student might be intently studying the chapter on medications to use in shock situations and runs across dopamine. He daydreams about a situation shortly after graduation from nursing school where the doctor turns to him and says, "This guy is on his way out. We need to get his pressure back up! Let's give him dopamine. Start a drip at 5 mcg/kg/min. Now!" The doctor turns away, confident her medication order will be implemented in the few minutes remaining before her patient dies. The pharmacology student, in his daydream, looks at the 250 mL bag containing 3.2 mg/mL of dopamine and the infusion pump and says, "Now what?"

# Math makes me sweat and twitch!

The brief scenarios described on the previous page mark the end points of the continuum, from fairly basic to pretty complex, giving the range of typical medication math situations encountered in daily nursing practice. Drug dosing and administration does involve conversions and calculations, and nurses do need to perform them accurately, but math is not always a comfortable area for us. This is true particularly for medication math since it uses strategies we learned long ago and don't easily recall.

**Don't panic:** The first and most important step to dealing with medication math is to learn a few basic definitions, measurements, and conversions.

The crucial first step and the focus of the rest of this lesson is to review systems of measurement or perhaps even to finally learn them for the first time. From a pharmacology point of view, it is not very complicated at all. We really are concerned only with the metric system, but we need to know the household measures to communicate with our patients.

### The mystery of household measures

We need to remember that household measures are not precise and are "second best" for dosage administration. They are, however, more familiar to our patients, so we must know common units and their relationship to systems used in healthcare. Memorize this table of common measures (italicized measurements are used more often in medication doses).

**Don't forget:**

## Household measures

**Liquid measures**

| | | |
|---|---|---|
| *1 tablespoon* | = | *3 teaspoons* |
| *1 fluid once* | = | *2 tablespoons  =  6 teaspoons* |
| 1 cup | = | 8 fluid ounces = 16 tablespoons = 48 teaspoons |
| 1 pint | = | 16 fluid ounces  = 2 cups |
| 1 quart | = | 2 pints |

**Weight measures**

| | | |
|---|---|---|
| *1 pound* | = | *16 ounces* |

## What is a microgram, anyway?

The apothecary's weight system was once used in medicine but has become an anachronism, now more confusing, and consequently dangerous, than useful. It included measurements such as 20 grains = 1 scruple, 3 scruples = 1 dram, 8 drams = 1 ounce, and 12 ounces = 1 pound. The casual reader immediately notices the differences between pound and ounces in this scheme vs. the household 16 ounces = 1 pound. (This is taken from the Avoirdupois classification, which is the English derived system we use in daily life). The Apothecary structure is interesting to historians but has little relevance for us today. Nevertheless, there is another arrangement that is supremely useful to us: the metric system.

The basic or root liquid metric unit is the liter (L). The basic or root mass (weight in terms of medications) unit is the gram (g).

Prefixes are added to modify the root. For example:

- Giga means 1,000,000,000

- Mega means 1,000,000

- Kilo means 1,000

- Deca means 10

- Liter/gram (the root) means 1

- Deci means 1/10

- Milli means 1/1000

- Mcg means 1/1,000,000

- Nano means 1/1,000,000,000

Think of some everyday examples to help you remember relative sizes. Many of us can relate to a typical Microsoft Word document as measured in KB (kilobytes) that we store in a folder containing MB (megabytes) and can load onto our GB (gigabyte) jump drive to take with us. Or perhaps we can remember that we have microscopes to look at very small things, not milliscopes, which will help us remember "milli" things are larger than "micro" things.

 **Tip:** The great thing about the metric system is that it is in multiples of 1000. If you remember the sequence of prefixes, the rest is easy.

We typically will use only a few of these prefixes in medication administration. So, the first step is to learn them.

**Tip:** In the past, cubic centimeters (cc) were used to describe liquid amounts in medicine. This unit no longer is customarily used because its abbreviation, cc, could be mistaken for 00 when handwritten. One cc in a medical context was equivalent to one mL.

Memorize the following table of metric items commonly used in pharmacology.

**Don't forget:**

| Common metric measurements | | |
|---|---|---|
| **Liquid measures** | | |
| 1000 mL | = | 1 liter |
| **Weight measures** | | |
| 1000 g | = | 1 kilogram |
| 1000 milligrams (mg) | = | 1 gram (g) |
| 1000 micrograms (mcg) | = | 1 milligram (mg) |

**Tip:** To remember the sequence for weight measures, remember "micro" as in microscope is smaller than "milli" as in millipede (you don't need a microscope to see a millipede!). Drug dealers want a "kilo" as in kilogram because it is bigger than a gram. Whether you are talking liters, meters, or grams, a unit of measure without any prefix is right in the middle.

## More on metric

Now, let's consider how you get from household to metric. If you know the measures listed in the previous tables and just a few simple conversions, you will have no difficulty getting from one system to the other. These are the only conversions you need to remember:

**Don't forget:**

## A few final measurements

- 1 kg = 2.2 lbs

- 1 tablespoon = 15 mL

- 1 teaspoon = 5 mL

- 1 fluid ounce = 30 mL

- 1 cm = 2.54 inches

There are a couple of other key concepts we need to learn as we look at conversions. The first is the idea of milliequivalents (mEq). This is a method of looking at substances in such a way that both their weight and chemical activity are considered. It is commonly used with electrolytes and some intravenous solutions that contain electrolytes.

You won't regularly be expected to do the calculation in day-to-day nursing practice, but you should have a basic awareness of how it is done. It is calculated by multiplying the milligrams per liter by the valence of the chemical and dividing by the molecular weight of the substance. From chemistry, you remember valence indicates the number of bonds a substance can form. Sodium has a valence of 1 and calcium has a valence of 2. Molecular weight (now also called molecular mass) is the mass or weight of one molecule of a substance and can be determined by the molecular weights and amounts of each kind of atom in the molecule.

To illustrate, because the electrolytes exist as the salt form of ionic molecules, the most common units used to describe the amount of the electrolytes are milliequivalents (mEq). A milliequivalent is a way to relate the weight of an electrolyte substance to its molecular weight. The benefit of using milliequivalents is that the term refers to the individual strength of each electrolyte in the salt form. For example, 10 mEq of sodium chloride refers to 10 mEq of sodium and 10 mEq of chloride. In this way, the dose of the elemental form of the sodium is clear. Sometimes the strengths of electrolytes are converted to a milligram amount (Corcoran).

**Tip:** Here's an example of where we will see mEq used: Sodium (Na) levels in the blood are measured in mEq of sodium per liter of blood for a normal range of 135–145 mEq/L.

Secondly, something we will touch more on later, is the idea of solutions that are expressed in percents. This refers to the mass of solute in grams per 100 mL of solution. To hold you over with an example, a 0.9% saline solution contains 0.9g of sodium chloride (NaCl) per 100ml of water.

## The sum of math

So, let's sum up this lesson:

- It's important to note that we all can learn (all of us managed to get through high school and some college courses)—we just need to have a system.

- The first, and one of the most important, things to learn in relation to accurate medication math calculation are a few basic definitions and conversions.

The last two lessons in Part 1 will examine getting and keeping our brains in shape and successful learning strategies.

## References

Corcoran, J. and Duncan, J. (2007). *Pediatric High-Alert Medications: Evidence-Based Safe Practices for Nursing Professional.* Marblehead, MA: HCPro, Inc.

Venes, D. and Thomas, C. (eds) (2001). *Taber's Cyclopedic Medical Dictionary.* Philadelphia: F.A. Davis Company.

# Chapter 3

# Keep up your learning hygiene

We need to pay just as much attention to our learning hygiene as we do to our physical hygiene. We keep our bodies clean (most of the time), and some of us work to keep in shape (sort of). Similar effort needs to be spent keeping our brain and body in condition to learn. You can't learn anything if basic physiologic needs are unmet or compromised.

Picture this: Your buddy Jake tells you on Thursday he can't hang with you on Sunday because he needs to study for Monday's pharm exam. However, he's okay with going out Saturday night. He decides to slack a bit because he works hard, full time at a job he doesn't really like to pay huge tuition bills so he can go to nursing school (which in itself seems to be a full-time job!) Jake works all day and then schleps off to school to study in the evening, every evening. Since he has no time for regular meals, he eats tons of donuts and fast food, and averages about five and a half to six hours of sleep each night.

Fast forward to Saturday. You both decide to relax, you've earned it. You watch a ballgame, enjoy more than medicinal amounts of snacks and beverages, then to the bar to rehash the game and meet a few friends. The first half of the Sunday study session morphs into a recovery day. Lots of snacks and beverages, a week's worth of sleep deprivation, and unabated day-to-day pressure and frustration all made studying futile.

The Monday morning pharm exam wasn't pretty . . .

# Boot camp for your brain

### Let's talk about sleep

Most people need six to eight hours of sleep daily to effectively function. The right amount of sleep for your body is not optional. Aside from being pretty goofy, people who lack sufficient sleep demonstrate clearly defined phenomena including:

- Daytime drowsiness

- Decreased ability to function

- Heightened sensitivity to pain

- Inability to concentrate

- Slowed reaction times

- Perceptual distortions

- Irritability

- Anxiety

This is far from an all-inclusive list. The lesson here is, since you know you need sleep, plan it. Protect your sleep time as much as you treasure your play time. Develop smart sleep habits.

 **Tip:** To help you get some much-needed shut-eye, try these four tips:

- Stick to a schedule as closely as you can.

- Avoid caffeine for several hours before sleep.

- Don't run a mile or eat a huge meal right before bed. Both disturb sleep.

- Save the bed for sleep—no reading in bed, no watching TV, etc. Condition your body to expect to sleep when it hits the bed.

### Hooray for exercise!

Physical activity is a great stress reliever, and dealing with stress allows us to direct more valuable energy to learning. Physiologic and psychological stresses confront us all. Someone coughs in our face, and we need to fight off disease. Our boss is a mini-dictator. All of our instructors think their class is the most important item in the universe. And don't get us started on the family issues. Sound familiar?

All of these trials—and even all of the great exciting things that happen to us—stimulate production of hormones, such as:

- Adrenocorticotropic hormone: alters immune function and water/electrolyte balance

- Vasopressin: raises blood pressure, causes fluid retention

- Growth hormone: affects protein/carbohydrate/fat metabolism and, ultimately, tissue repair

- Thyrotropic hormone: affects basal metabolic rate

- Gonadotropins: prolonged effect includes decreased libido and impotence

These substances are responsible for the "fight or flight" response you've heard of in the past. This reaction is a great thing during life-threatening emergencies, but if prolonged, it decreases our immune system effectiveness, elevates the glucose and fat content in our blood, diminishes our sexual functioning, and stresses our cardiovascular system among other things.

DAILY (sorry for yelling, but it is important) exercise moderates the effects of prolonged stress, makes you feel better, increases your energy and ability to cope, and, most importantly for us, dramatically increases your ability to concentrate and learn!

 **Don't forget:** Thirty to forty-five minutes of exercise a day earns colossal dividends.

You want to select types of exercise that appeal to you and that strengthen, increase flexibility, and enhance cardiovascular functioning. Running, biking, and swimming are obvious choices. Less intuitive options include yoga (one of the best!) and brisk walking. Your school or work may have a fitness center where you can use equipment and receive guidance at a reduced rate.

One easy and convenient method to boost your activity is to add steps to your day:

- Take the stairs instead of the elevator

- Park in the parking spot furthest from the entrance rather than close by

- Go talk to someone at work instead of calling or e-mailing, as it helps build relationships

- Walk during work breaks

- Walk, don't drive, whenever possible

- Wear a pedometer to measure your progress

### It's chow time!

**Don't forget:** Nutrition is vital!

You would think this is a no-brainer, but inadequate nutrition remains a powerful influence on student performance. Food fuels learning! Choose to maximize the benefits you can obtain from eating well. First, there is the matter of calories: Ensure you get an adequate amount but not too much. The first step is to calculate your basic metabolic rate (BMR) using the appropriate formula below:

- Women: BMR = 655 + (4.35 x weight in pounds) + (4.7 x height in inches) - (4.7 x age in years)

- Men: BMR = 66 + (6.23 x weight in pounds) + (12.7 x height in inches) - (6.8 x age in years)

The next stage is to calculate your required calories using the Harris Benedict Equation:

1. If you are sedentary (little or no exercise), calorie calculation = BMR x 1.2

2. If you are lightly active (light exercise/sports 1–3 days/week), calorie calculation = BMR x 1.375

3. If you are moderately active (moderate exercise/sports 3–5 days/week), calorie calculation = BMR x 1.55

4. If you are very active (hard exercise/sports 6–7 days a week), calorie calculation = BMR x 1.725

5. If you are extra active (very hard exercise/sports and a physical job or 2x training), calorie-calculation = BMR x 1.9

After you have calculated the calories, stick to it! You can find reliable online sources that describe the calorie content of common foods. Be sure you eat enough to meet your needs each day. Sufficient calories are crucial, but so is the variety of food.

Be sure you eat adequate protein (meats, beans, whole grains) for tissue repair and energy, carbohydrates for quick energy, and vitamins and minerals to catalyze physiological reactions. If your diet isn't diverse and rich in fresh fruits and produce, taking a multivitamin can't hurt. Finally, drink water—lots of it: eight 8-ounce glasses each day, and more if you are sweating. This water is in place of soda, juices, caffeinated drinks, and alcoholic beverages.

## Keep it all in balance

This can be a difficult time for you as you may be juggling work, family, and school obligations. Take a few moments to sit down and consider your schedule. It is easy to become overloaded and develop a sense of frustration and helplessness, so take control!

Make a list of things that are important to you and rank them. I'm sure pharmacology is at the top of your list . . . ahem, well, just wishful thinking on my part. You cannot reasonably hope to do all things for you and everyone else all the time (remember what we learned about sleep deprivation?). Create a list of achievable expectations that balance your needs and obligations.

Going to school and doing well means you have to give something up or delay it for the duration—perhaps cutting back on TV, reducing some hobby time, or temporarily limiting volunteer commitments. It is more gratifying for most people to shrink the scope of what they do and continue to perform well than to add more tasks and have performance suffer overall. Maintain "you" time. You will be happier and learn better if you acknowledge the need for family time and fun moments—schedule them and make sure you indulge! Then, study time will be free of resentment and feelings of oppression.

## So, you're feeling a bit stressed?

As students and new graduates, you know nurses are fascinating multidimensional beings. Although it is impossible to delineate the boundaries in any definitive way, we exist in physical/physiological, cognitive (thinking), affective (mood), and spiritual worlds.

We devoted some time to our physical health and will examine thinking in the next lesson, so let's finish up this class by mulling over other perspectives.

First, we've already seen how stress builds up, and we came to realize that exercise will help. Another useful tool is to regularly indulge (because it really is an enjoyable treat) in structured and scheduled relaxation exercises. Here's an easy and wonderfully effective technique to try.

## Take a breath

We all breathe on a somewhat regular basis without giving the process any thought. Read through these steps, and then give it a try.

1. Find a quiet comfortable place to sit or lie down. Get yourself as comfortable as you can without going to sleep.

2. Stretch your arms and legs and jaw (it may stimulate a yawn).

3. Allow yourself to take this time for you, to leave all cares and concerns behind for these few moments.

4. Close your eyes. Take a slow, deep breath in through your nose feeling the air swirl and make its way deep into your lungs.

5. Don't purposely slow your breathing; allow it to find its own pace and rhythm. With each exhalation, you will feel more at ease and more relaxed. Concentrate on your breath.

6. As extraneous thoughts enter your mind, acknowledge them and gently nudge them away like a helium-filled balloon. Let them drift away from you.

7. Just breathe.

8. When it feels right, think about opening your eyes and slowly rolling your shoulders and stretching your neck. Now, slowly open your eyes while remembering how relaxed you feel.

This is most effective if you do it for approximately 20–25 minutes twice a day. You can also use this exercise to help you gain energy and focus, yet remain relaxed before an exam. Just take a few minutes to get in your zone and replenish your body with a few deep oxygen-rich breaths!

## We're in this together

We are social creatures and want/need to maintain linkages with others on various levels. Anytime we think we are unique individuals, we just need to examine our behavior. We dress alike, keep similar schedules, join clubs, gather at sports arenas, respond to the same ads on TV, and resonate to the same political speeches (is there really that much substantive difference between parties and candidates?). We are no more the absolutely unique creatures we imagine ourselves than specific animals in a flock of penguins or a herd of wildebeests. That is a good thing! It means we are not alone.

Maintain your relationships. Nurture them as if you were weeding and fertilizing a garden. These people will give you the consolation and support you may need if you become discouraged. You can't help but learn when you've got people rooting for you!

Okay, now that we are all suitably nourished, exercised to an exquisite level of buffness, have arranged our priorities, have reached absolute relaxation, and have established our social supports, it's a perfect time to learn how to learn!

## References

Bellisle, F. (2001). "Glucose and mental performance." *The British Journal of Nutrition,* 86(2), 117-8.

"BMI Calculator: BMR Formula." Available at *www.bmi-calculator.net/ bmr-calculator/bmr-formula.php.* Accessed November 8, 2007.

"BMI Calculator: Harris Benedict Equation." Available at *www.bmi-calculator.net/ bmr-calculator/harris-benedict-equation.* Accessed November 8, 2007.

Budilovsky, J. and Adamson, E. (2001). *The Complete Idiot's Guide to Yoga* (2nd ed.) Indianapolis: Alpha Books

Dani, J., Burrill, C., and Demmig-Adams, B. (2005). "The remarkable role of nutrition in learning and behaviour." *Nutrition and Food Science,* 35(3/4), 258-263.

Myers, T. (editor). 2006. *Mosby's Dictionary of Medicine, Nursing & Health Professions.* (7th ed.) St. Louis: Elsevier.

Seyler, D. (1984). *Read, Reason, Write.* New York: Random House

Sprenger, M. (1999). *Learning and Memory: The Brain in Action.* Alexandria, Va.: Association for Supervision and Curriculum Development.

Townsend, M. (2006). *Psychiatric Mental Health Nursing: Concepts of Care in Evidence-Based Practice* (5th ed.) Philadelphia: FA Davis Company.

# Chapter 4

# Go on, dive right in . . .

We are almost ready to take the plunge. This lesson, we'll stay in the shallow end with some learning tips. Remember, don't leave learning to chance— have a plan and use proven methods!

## Know thyself

Lots of philosophers, sages, wits, and late-night comics have suggested we ought to "know" ourselves. The Roman philosopher and emperor Marcus Aurelius took it a step further: "Look well into thyself; there is a source of strength which will always spring up if thou wilt always look there." There is a lot of truth in that. You are your best resource, your best teacher, and your best cheerleader. You will be successful in pharmacology and as a practicing nurse if you know yourself—strengths, weaknesses, natural tendencies, inclinations—and effectively use that self-knowledge. Take a few moments to do a self-awareness inventory and ask yourself:

- At what time of day am I most alert?

- Do I learn best by doing, reading, hearing, or seeing?

- What strategies have helped me learn in the past?

- How much willpower and motivation do I have?

- Do I see myself as a quick or slow learner?

Other questions may occur to you, but the point is to assess first, analyze your data next, and come up with a plan last. Then, try out your interventions and examine the results. Those of you in nursing school will recognize this as the basic nursing process. If you are not taking nursing classes but learn this now, it is one less thing to learn later!

Let's look at some tried and true strategies that will help make this course a success.

## Chunk it, memorize it, and learn it

Try these ideas to organize and process information:

- Learn to read. This isn't meant to be offensive, but it's a basic strategy we don't uniformly employ.

- Prepare to become part of the author's audience—in this case, as a student. Be a student, meaning inquisitive, interested, and anxious to learn.

- Read slowly, as slow as you need to get through the material and understand it. Look up words you don't know as you go along. Make flash cards of new words. Time is needed here.

- Make notes as you read. It is guaranteed to help you remember.

- Read each section more than once, preferably several days apart.

**Use bulletin boards or posters.** Most of the time, your class content will be organized into units or chapters. How great is that? The entire course is already organized into chunks. Now, just make a poster or bulletin board of each chunk as you go along. Don't worry about how the poster looks, since only you will see it. Use one of those big, 2x3 foot pads of cheap paper from an art supply or teaching store. Put content in word balloons or weird shapes and link it together with colored, silly, swirled arrows. Have some fun. When you try to recall the information later on, you will actually "see" the picture and REMEMBER (sorry for shouting)!

**Perform the material.** Acting isn't necessarily everyone's reason to live, but for those of us who like it, act out the lesson. Be the vasoconstrictive alpha 1 receptor, for example, and act out what happens with Afrin nasal spray (Afrin is an alpha adrenergic agonist that causes constriction of blood vessels to reduce swelling and congestion). If you are too inhibited, create an image in your mind of some other poor soul doing the acting. When you want to remember the material, just replay the scene. It works!

**Try memory pegs and mnemonics.** These are crutches to help you remember. Don't be afraid to use these memory assistants!

Pegs are common words or images that you "peg" your information to. For example:

- 1=sun

- 2=blue

- 3=tree

- 4=shore

. . . and so on.

This rhyming peg is a great way to remember numbers. Create your own system that uses words or images appealing to you—things you don't have to work at remembering—and then use your peg to help you stun people with your memory.

Mnemonics are another fascinating tool. They are words we create by using the first letters of the facts we need to learn. Later on, we can use the word to retrieve the data.

Here is one of my favorites: ABBA. Here's the secret: To me, ABBA means alpha 1 / beta 1/ beta 2/ alpha 2. These are the peripheral nervous system receptors. When I say ABBA (which used to be a musical group—think "Dancing Queen"—so it is easy to remember), this is what floods into my head:

- There are four kinds of peripheral nerve receptors

- Alpha 1 is important (at the beginning of ABBA), and lots of drugs affect this to promote or inhibit vasoconstriction

- Beta 1 is important (first B in ABBA) and refers to the heart since beta 1 = 1 heart

- Beta 2 is important (second B in ABBA) and refers to the lungs since beta 2 = 2 lungs

- Alpha 2 exists, but is not important in the periphery since it comes at the end of ABBA

Feel free to use it, and create your own mnemonics using words important to you.

## More ways to ingrain ideas in your brain

 **Tip:** Don't even try to memorize every drug separately. People who can do that have a special gift!

Drugs are sorted into classes or related groups, such as beta blockers, calcium channel blockers, benzodiazepines, etc. One of the cool things about pharmacology is, generally speaking, all beta blockers behave in a similar fashion, as do members of other drug classifications. So, let's consider this list:

- Pindolol

- Propranolol

- Sotalol

- Timolol

- Metoprolol

We would note a certain similarity in the last syllable of each and suspect they belong to the same family. Learn the characteristics of the family, and then just study the small differences between the members. That road is a whole lot easier to travel down.

### Lecturing to the dog and other learning miracles

- Be the teacher. We all, generally speaking, want to like and think well of ourselves. We try to make ourselves feel good. So we unconsciously tend to study stuff we know because when we remember it, we feel good. What's the tip here? Pretend you are the teacher.

  Deliver the week's lecture(s) to your dog or cat or kid (if they can be securely restrained). You will prattle on and on but eventually will get stuck. The information you get stuck on is the only stuff you need to study. Don't put any effort into rehashing the things you've already learned other than quick periodic run-throughs to keep it cemented and to deepen the memory groove. Do focus most of your energy on the areas you are less sure about; your lectures will invariably identify them for you.

- Make use of automatic memory. This is memory that, eventually, you don't have to think about. Quick, what's your phone number? See, you can just rattle it off automatically. Flash cards will help you develop automatic memory, but don't make a card for everything. (It really may not help to have 500 or so for each chapter.) But do make one for each important concept, drug class, individual drug, and so on.

- Do some storytelling. There once was a wonderful opera singer (pretty, too) who became so anxious whenever she went onstage that she would feel her heart pounding and break into a cold sweat. Sometimes she even had to run offstage. Her doctor told her not to worry. "I shall give thee the magical propranolol," he said. The singer took it, her heart stopped pounding, and she no longer sweated. It worked fine for a time, but as she grew more famous and sang several shows daily, she used more and more of the magical propranolol. Then, one day she wheezed so much that she squeaked when she sang and her heart began to beat only two times per minute. She fell down. Every time she sat up to sing, her blood pressure plummeted and she passed out after three notes. It was a tediously long concert.

    Make up stories like the one above to give you a picture of the information, a kind of entertaining (if they are good stories) peg. The story above will help me remember that a nonselective beta blocker can be used to treat an anxiety disorder such as stage fright but may cause asthma attacks in susceptible people, bradycardia (slow heart rate), and hypotension (abnormally low blood pressure).

## The down and dirty about cramming

Don't do it! The only way to actually learn is through repetition, and devoting time and energy DAILY (sorry for shouting again). Even 15 or 20 minutes a day of focused effort will pay off better than pulling an all-nighter.

That being said, did you ever wonder how actors in a TV drama learn new scenes every week? They cram! It does work! Life happens; sometimes our best intentions can't be carried out, and we need to cram. If you are up against a wall and have to cram, use all of the tools listed above: pegs, mnemonics, posters, etc.

 **Tip:** If you have to cram, eat high energy foods (protein), drink lots of water, drink small amounts of caffeine (larger amounts are counterproductive), take cat naps, and take frequent short breaks.

You will remember a lot of the information—for less than a day. Cramming can be a useful tool, but ultimately you will put nothing in long-term memory if cramming is all you do.

## Don't do it alone

We are social creatures for the most part. Though hitting the books with someone doesn't take the place of frequent solitary study, it is a useful adjunct and can be a valuable strategy. The benefits include:

- Having someone urge us on when we would just as soon put it off until tomorrow.

- Our partner(s) often give us a new perspective and prevent us from over-looking important information.

- Trying to explain something to someone else really helps us see if we understand it.

- Misery loves company. It often is truly a comfort to know we are not alone and are supported. This, in turn, reduces our frustration and improves our learning.

 **Don't forget:** Learning requires time and a plan. Daily study periods using specific strategies will guarantee success!

Now that we are prepared to learn, let's move on to the good stuff: the pharmacology lessons in Part 2.

## References

Lehne, R. (2007). *Pharmacology for Nursing Care* 6th ed. St. Louis: Saunders.

Seyler, D. (1984). *Read, Reason, Write.* New York: Random House.

Sprenger M. (1999) *Learning and Memory: The Brain in Action.* Alexandria, VA.: Association for Supervision and Curriculum Development.

# Part two

Unofficial medications, pharmacokinetics, the five rights, and the three checks are just some of the topics we'll touch on in this section. Take your time, learn them, and you'll soon find yourself at the head of the class.

# Chapter 5

# The down low on drugs

 **Did you know:** Pharmaceuticals are big business. The top 10 companies, in terms of sales, had total profits of $39,780,689,350 in 2006 (Committee on Government Reform). That is not what they sold; it is what they made after paying all of their costs!

Stroll up and down the aisles of your local drug store, and notice how many products are available. Prescribed and over-the-counter medications have made a spectacular impact on our collective health and ease the symptoms of non-life-threatening but annoying maladies. As we continue our pharmacology class, let's reflect on what exactly we mean by medications or drugs and attempt to establish the boundaries of their role.

For the sake of simplicity and clarity, we are going to choose to define drugs as *substances that affect processes in living beings* and medications as *drugs purposely given to treat disease or alleviate symptoms* (Lehne). These indicate we are thinking about both effect and purpose. Examples of drugs could include things such as the beta-carotene in carrots and the pollutants we inhale from the factory down the road, and medications—such as penicillin and aspirin—that initially leap to mind.

We've established what medications are, so now let's take on the tough question: How are they appropriately used?

**Don't forget:** Medications are not a way for us to avoid making hard life-style decisions!

One of your roles as a nurse is to teach. We give our patients the information they need to assume responsibility for their own health and wellness. Part of that task is to teach medication use as maximizing—but not replacing—the benefits achieved by a healthy lifestyle. For example, there has been a massive increase in obesity rates in the United States.

**Did you know:** Fifteen percent of Americans aged 20 to 74 years were obese in 1980. By 2004, the rate increased to 33%. There also was a rise in childhood (6–11 years) obesity from approximately 16% to 19% in that time frame (Centers for Disease Control and Prevention, Overweight).

These substantially increasing rates should concern us because of obesity's known influence on health. Being overweight or obese sets the stage for conditions such as:

- Hypertension (27% of Americans are hypertensive) (Centers for Disease Control and Prevention, Hypertension)

- Dyslipidemia (for example, high total cholesterol or high levels of triglycerides)

- Type 2 diabetes

- Coronary heart disease

- Stroke

- Gallbladder disease

- Osteoarthritis

- Sleep apnea and respiratory problems

- Some cancers (endometrial, breast, and colon)

Treatment of the diseases listed above collectively account for nearly all of the most commonly prescribed medications (Centers for Disease Control and Prevention, Hypertension). Obesity certainly is not the only cause for these conditions, but it should be clear to us that maintaining a normal weight reduces the risk of developing these diseases with the resultant need for treatment. Other lifestyle issues include smoking, excess alcohol consumption, and choices related to personal safety such as seat belts, safe sex practices, and so on. Remember, just because you are on a drug to lower blood cholesterol, it doesn't mean you can eat that whole deep-dish, double-cheese, extra-everything pizza for a snack without health consequences.

## Official vs. unofficial medications

We all, perhaps, have a general sense of what official medications are. We would identify them as the antibiotic our doctor (or nurse practitioner) prescribes for that infection. Or the prescription pain medication. Or the blood pressure pill. Or the insulin shot for diabetes, etc. We think of these substances as potentially risky and requiring an expert's care in determining need and appropriate dosage. We would be accurate.

The experienced care provider has to sort through a lot of possible and similar diagnoses before selecting the right therapy because inappropriate treatment could lead to death or permanent disability. Also, many prescription drugs have only a slender difference in the dose required to be effective, and it's one that could cause illness or death. These official medicines have great potential to harm as well as aid us.

Now, how many times have you or someone you know developed a case of the runny nose sniffles, a sore back, or an annoying cough and went to the local mini-mart or drug store to pick up a little something for relief? Most of us would readily admit we've used nonprescription remedies. That's why they are available, right?

Can we take a quick poll of our class? All of you who have really read all of the small print on the side of those over-the-counter (OTC) medication boxes or package inserts, raise your hands. Thought so—only a few of you! I can hear some in the class asking: "What's the issue? They're not real medicines, and they're harmless, aren't they?" The answer is they are real medicines, and they may or may not be safe. OTC medications tend to be those with proven effectiveness that have not hurt large numbers of people when taken as directed. Often, they began as prescription-only drugs.

It wasn't too long ago that ibuprofen (Motrin®, Advil®, etc.), cimetidine (Tagamet®), and loratadine (Claritin®) were available only by prescription. But all eventually became OTC medications, meaning safe and effective for use based on OTC labeling and without the assistance of a professional.

The U.S. Food and Drug Administration (FDA, a government regulatory agency) often rightly agrees. That being said, would it surprise you to learn that acetaminophen, the active ingredient in Tylenol® and other preparations, causes more cases of liver failure than drinking alcoholic beverages? Most of those instances stem from improper use and occur in people who *didn't read the fine print on the box*. What would you say if you learned that cimetidine, the active ingredient in Tagamet®, can cause cognitive or thinking changes in elderly people that looks like Alzheimer's disease despite being taken as directed? The lesson for us is that OTC preparations are medicines with all the benefits and possible hazards associated with "official" medicines.

**Watch out:** Always remember that any medicine with good effects can potentially produce harmful effects!

## Medicines vs. natural remedies

We are in a time of transition. For most of the last century, proponents and practitioners of organized medicine genuinely regarded themselves as the ultimate healthcare authorities and protectors of the public health and welfare. Herbs, meditation, therapeutic touch, chiropractic medicine, acupressure and acupuncture, and other modalities all were classified as unproven and probably ineffective *alternative* treatments. Despite the bad press, ill people who used them often improved—sometimes after conventional treatments failed. The disputes between proponents and opponents of alternative treatments have become less strident and polarized in recent years, and enough research has been conducted demonstrating effectiveness to warrant a change in name and reputation.

Alternative treatments now are known by the more inclusive title *complementary therapy* and have gained legitimacy.

**Did you know:** Thirty-six percent of Americans, according to a National Institutes of Health survey, use forms of complementary therapy to supplement traditional approaches (National Institutes of Health).

We can expect many of our patients to be using complementary remedies, including herbs, vitamins, spices, or other "natural" substances. Sometimes, our patients are seeing skilled and educated complementary providers. Some of our clients select their own remedies based on word of mouth from friends or relatives. Often people use them because lack of insurance or resources limits access to healthcare. Whatever the motivation, we need to know (and to teach our patients):

- "Natural" isn't synonymous with safe. We've already learned that every-thing that has a good effect has possible adverse effects.

- Complementary remedies such as herbs and vitamins can interact with prescribed conventional medications and potentially worsen health.

- Herbs and other complementary remedies are regulated by the FDA as food products and are checked only for things such as contaminants and adulterants (insect parts, dirt, etc.) and not for levels of effective ingredi-ents, for example.

- Errors associated with self-diagnosing have real dangers whether we take "real medicines" or "natural remedies."

## A quick Rx review

Let's wrap up this lesson. We've learned that anything that affects the pro-cesses going on in our bodies can be considered drugs, and drugs that are given to treat disease or address symptoms are termed medications. We've also come to know the only difference between "official" prescribed medi-cations and "unofficial" OTC meds is the latter tend to be more suited for self-diagnosed conditions and have a proven safety track record if appropri-ately used. We now understand natural or complementary medicines can be useful but present some concerns of their own. Perhaps most importantly, we have come to know that any medication with good or desired effects can have potential adverse effects and shouldn't be used without also looking at lifestyle changes.

Now, take a deep breath. We need to learn all about drug names!

## References

"Hypertension Statistics." Centers for Disease Control and Prevention. Available at *www.cdc.gov/nchs/data/hus/hus06.pdf#069*. Accessed November 9, 2007.

Lehne, R. (2007). *Pharmacology for Nursing Care*, 6th ed. St. Louis: Elsevier.

"Overweight and Obesity." Centers for Disease Control and Prevention. Available at *www.cdc.gov/nccdphp/dnpa/obesity*. Accessed November 9, 2007.

"Pharmaceutical industry profits increase by over $8 billion after Medicare drug plan goes into effect." Committee on Government Reform. Available at *http://oversight.house.gov/documents/20060919115623-70677.pdf*. Accessed November 10, 2007.

"The use of complementary and alternative medicine in the United States." National Center for Complementary and Alternative Medicine, National Institutes of Health. Available at *http://nccam.nih.gov/news/camsurvey_fs1.htm*. Accessed November 10, 2007.

# Chapter 6

# How are drugs named? Knowing nomenclature!

Don't drug names seem confusing? Consider Vasotec®. It is a drug prescribed to treat hypertension, reduce systemic vascular resistance, and increase cardiac output in patients with heart failure. It can also inhibit development of heart failure in patients with left ventricular dysfunction. Who'd guess that from Vasotec® or even another of its names, enalapril? Let's spend a few minutes in this lesson sorting out drug names. What we are interested in finding is a name that is descriptive, unique, and easy to remember.

## Cue the chemical names

There is a certain comfort to chemical names because of their precision. Chemical names plainly describe the structure of a given medication. There is no metaphysical angst about what the name means, no confusion as to its derivation, and utterly no chance of mistaking it for something else. Tell the name to a chemist, and he or she will know exactly what you mean. Enalapril maleate, also known as Vasotec®, is chemically described as (S)-1-[N-[1-(ethoxycarbonyl)-3-phenylpropyl]-L-alanyl]-L-proline, (Z)-2-butene-dioate salt (1:1). We can be even more tediously explicit and sketch its likeness (Drug InfoNet):

## Figure 1: Chemical description of enalapril maleate

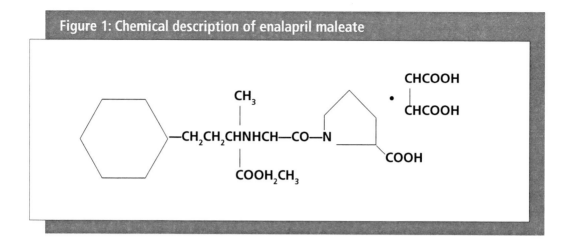

Don't you just adore the stunning symmetry between the coy phenol group and the vigorous carboxylic salt? Enough already! But can you see yourself toddling off to the drug store and saying, "My nurse practitioner tells me I need to take some ess dash one dash paragraph capital 'n' subparagraph one dash ethoxycarbonyl . . . "? We need another alternative. Thankfully, we have brand names.

## Bring on the brand (or trade) names

How did Coca-Cola get its name? How about Mountain Dew? Can anyone fail to recognize McDonald's or not know the name refers to hamburgers and fries, not old farmers in kilts? Companies want their product to be known and sought, which we call brand recognition.

It's the same in the drug world. Pharmaceutical companies, at great expense, develop medications and need to recoup their investments. If a couple of companies develop similar drugs with comparable actions and effects, each producer feels pressure to garner a larger market share to maximize profits. The need arises for an easy-to-remember, catchy, attractive, descriptive name linking it to the desired market. The poorly chosen brand will doom a product, so naming isn't done whimsically. Great effort is expended to create the resonant evocative name.

If you were to hear "the little purple pill," you would almost certainly recognize it as an effective remedy for gastroesophageal reflux disease. It's interesting to note studies suggest that Nexium® may be no more effective than other cheaper nonprescription medications including one made by the same company (Elliot and Ives).

Brand names are proprietary names and can't be used by any other company. New drugs themselves are patent-protected by a convoluted process and can't be produced by any other manufacturer until the patent protection expires. When competing companies are able to make the drug, each entity must create its own brand name. This explains why ibuprofen can be bought as Advil®, Amersol®, Motrin®, Children's Motrin®, Ibuprin®, Mediprin®, Nuprin®, Pediaprofen®, Pamprin-IB®, Rufen®, and Trendar®. It looks like brand names are not the answer to our problems either.

## Give generic names a try

Wouldn't it be great if each drug had one short, memorable, descriptive name that would give you a hint of its relationship with other medications? There is a group named the United States Adopted Names Council that aspires to do just that. It is an organization jointly sponsored by the American Medical Association (AMA), the United States Pharmacopeial Convention, and the American Pharmaceutical Association, whose aim is to contribute to a standard global drug nomenclature (naming system).

The council creates and assigns unique generic names to new pharmaceuticals marketed in the United States. The goal is to make them simple and informative. Well, look at some of these newly assigned generic names: *agatolimod sodium* (anticancer), *amrubicin hydrochloride* (antineoplastic), *laromustine* (antileukemic), *ropinirole* (Parkinson's disease and restless leg syndrome), *sergliflozin etabonate* (type 2 diabetes), *sorafenib* (treatment of cancer), *sorafenib tosylate* (treatment of cancer), and *veltuzumab* (treatment of non-Hodgkin's lymphoma). Easy, simple, informative . . . what are we missing here?

All jests aside, let's look at the first drug, agatolimod, which is a newly named anticancer medication. Although at first blush agatolimod doesn't seem to be an uncomplicated and straightforward name, compare it with the chemical name: P-thiothymidaylyl5'-(3'→5')-2'-deoxy-P-thiocytidylyl-(3'→5')2'-deoxy-P-thioguanylyl-(3'→5')-P-thiothymidylyl-(3'→5')-2'deoxy-P-thio-cytidylyl-(3'→5')-2'-deoxy-P-thiothymidyly-(3'→5')-P-thiothymidylyl-(3'→5')- . . . goes on for six more incredibly detailed lines . . . tricosasodium salt. That doesn't exactly roll effortlessly off one's tongue either!

Let's go back to our earlier example, enalapril. It belongs to a class of drugs called angiotensin converting enzyme inhibitors, or ACE inhibitors. Other members of that class include:

- Captopril

- Fosinopril

- Lisinopril

- Moexipril

- Perindopril

- Quinapril

- Ramipril

- Trandolapril

Anyone see a pattern here? The suffix points toward a shared relationship and effect while the root connotes distinctive characteristics. Generic seems like the way to go!

 **Tip:** The generic names, without a doubt, are less cumbersome than the chemical names and more descriptive than brand names.

## Applying our knowledge to a patient

Picture this. You are a home-care nurse (one who makes house calls like doctors did in the old days), and you have a patient named Mabel. You saw her on Wednesday, found she had high blood pressure and a rapid pulse, so you got her in to see her cardiologist. On Friday, you went to check on Mabel. She tells you the doctor prescribed Calan®, and she asks you about it. You teach her what it is for and what to watch out for because you know that any medication that has good effects also has potential adverse effects. You also tell her you will return on Monday to see how she is.

On Monday, you return and find Mabel's heart rate to be in the 40s (way too low for her) and her blood pressure to be 92/38 (way too low for her). She is also nauseated, constipated, dizzy, and has a severe headache. Her feet and lower legs are swollen, so she plainly is not doing well. While you wait for the ambulance, she tells you, "I still didn't feel good after you left on Friday, so I drove to the emergency room. They checked me over and gave me a prescription for Isoptin®. On Saturday, I still felt pretty bad so I went to the other hospital emergency room, and they gave me a prescription for vera-pamil. I took all of my medicines just like they told me to. I don't understand what happened to me."

What do you think happened? You guessed it. Well done! Verapamil is a generic name, and Isoptin® and Calan® are proprietary or brand names—all for the same medication. Mabel neglected to tell Saturday's emergency department doctor about the Thursday physician visit. She also failed to tell the Sunday emergency room staff members about either of the earlier doctors and prescriptions. Mabel nearly died.

Other problems, like the true story just described, have arisen. Sometimes the names are just too close. Consider these examples:

- An eight-year-old died after receiving morphine (opioid pain reliever) instead of methylphenidate (stimulant for Attention Deficit Hyperactivity Disorder)

- A 19-year-old man nearly died after being given clozapine (antipsychotic) instead of olanzapine (another antipsychotic) (Rados)

Some brand names are mistaken for other brand names. Sometimes brand names are confused with generics, and sometimes, even some generics are mistaken for other generics.

## So, what do I need to know?

Here's where the rubber hits the road as far as drug names go. As a nurse, you need to know:

- The generic and common brand names for all medications frequently used in your area of practice

- How to look up any unfamiliar medication prior to administering it

And, as a patient advocate, you must teach those under your care:

- To learn the generic and brand (if taking a name-brand drug) names of their medications or at least keep a current list of medications handy

- To fill prescriptions at just one pharmacy to decrease risk of duplication or interactions

# References

Elliot, S. and Ives, N. "US: Questions on the $3.8 Billion Drug Ad Business," *New York Times*, October 13, 2004, found on CorpWatch: Holding Corporations Accountable. Available at *www.corpwatch.org/article.php?id=11572*. Accessed November 10, 2007.

Rados, C. "Drug Name Confusion: Preventing Medication Errors." MedicineNet.com. Available at *www.medicinenet.com/script/main/art.asp?articlekey=53208*. Accessed November 10, 2007.

"United States Adopted Names." American Medical Association. Available at *www.ama-assn.org/ama/pub/category/2956.html*. Accessed November 10, 2007.

"Vasotec Package Insert." Drug InfoNet. Available at *www.druginfonet.com/index.php?pageID=vasotec.htm*. Accessed November 10, 2007.

Wilson, B., Shannon, M., Shields, K., and Stang, C. (2007). *Nurse's Drug Guide 2007*. Upper Saddle River, New Jersey: Prentice Hall.

# Chapter 7

# The five rights and three checks: We're not obsessive— we're just nurses!

In mental health nursing, we encounter people plagued with anxiety related to obsessive and intrusive thoughts. The anxiety is relieved only by performing an action. For example, someone may experience a pervasive fear of becoming contaminated somehow, and the anxiety abates only after hand washing. The unfortunate person may feel compelled to wash hundreds of times a day. We would call that anxiety maladaptive because it interferes with normal functioning and creates distress.

In contrast, in this lesson, we are going to create a healthy sense of anxiety and instill some adaptive compulsions. Your new obsessive-compulsive behaviors will actually relieve your overall anxiety and grant you some confidence in your competence at medication administration. This isn't the formal math lesson, but let's do a quick calculation or two.

## Laying a foundation

First, let's lay out some background data: A typical day-shift nurse on a medical surgical unit may have six patients depending on the region of the country. Let's say each patient receives six medications three times during the 12-hour day shift (a conservative estimate). Let's also assume the nurse works six shifts every two weeks. How many medications does the nurse pass each week? How about each year?

Turn those gears in your head: X drug doses/week = 6 patients x 4 meds/pass x 3 passes/day x 3 days/week = 216 drug doses/week or 10,800 drug doses/ year (allowing two weeks vacation—everyone needs vacation!).

**Watch out:** Now the scary part. Let's say you pass the meds perfectly 99% of the time. That means you could potentially injure or kill 108 patients a year! See for yourself: 10,800 drug doses/year x 0.01 errors = 108 drug errors per year.

Most patients survive errors in hospitals, but in an important study in 1999, the Institute of Medicine (IOM) estimated that 100,000 people died each year from assorted errors. More recent sources put the number closer to 195,000 (Medical News Today). The National Academy of Sciences, of which the IOM is one of four partners, continues to monitor current research and reports that 400,000 preventable drug injuries occur each year in hospitals plus another 800,000 in extended-care facilities (National Academies of Science).

**Don't panic:** If you learn and scrupulously follow the "five rights" system, your patients will be safe. This is obsessive in a good way!

## Right on with the five rights

Here are the five rights of medication administration (no particular order is needed):

**Patient:** It seems silly to actually say out loud we need to confirm our patient's identity, doesn't it? Believe this: Sometimes patients are so ill or disoriented, they actually respond to the wrong name. Professional nurses know this and always confirm the patient's identity three ways:

- Asking the patient (a reliable family member may also identify the client).

- Looking at the patient's name band (placed on the wrist when the patient is admitted); some facilities require scanning the bar code on the wrist band.

- Asking the person his/her birth date.

**Medication:** We already looked at confusion that sometimes occurs due to drug names. This is a great occasion to recheck and be completely convinced this is the correct drug. Ask:

- Is this the medication the doctor prescribed?

- Does this medication make sense, given the client's disease and condition?

**Dose:** Prescribing medications is beyond our scope of practice, but nurses must know (or look up when in doubt) safe and therapeutic doses. Ask:

- Is this the standard dose?

- Are there circumstances that indicate the dose should be modified?

  - Age? Elders often require lower doses of some medications.

  - Body size? Some medications are dosed in micrograms per kilogram of body weight.

  - Abnormal physical assessment findings? A medication to lower blood pressure should not be administered if the client's blood pressure already is too low.

  - Abnormal laboratory findings? It may not be appropriate to give a potassium supplement if the client's potassium blood level is elevated.

  - Abnormal organ function? Someone with impaired liver or kidney function may need lower doses of common medications.

  - Any other relevant concerns? For example, as a nurse, you should not administer medicines to control high blood pressure immediately prior to renal dialysis.

**Time:** Are you giving the drug at the right time?

- For example, is it due at 9 p.m., and are you preparing to give it at 9 a.m.?

- Does the medicine need to be given with or without food? For example, thyroid hormone is supposed to be given one hour before breakfast.

**Route:** Are you administering an oral medication orally? Are you administering an intravenous medication through an intravenous line?

## Don't forget the three checks!

The rule is to check, recheck, and recheck again whether you are complying with the five rights.

1.  The first check is when we pull the medications or retrieve them from automated dispensing machine (sometimes called the Pyxis), the medication drawer, or whatever system is in place at a given institution.

2.  The second check is when we are preparing the medications for administration.

3.  The final check occurs at the patient's bedside just before we give the medications. This is also an outstanding opportunity to teach the patient about the medicines.

**Don't forget:** Skilled and safe nurses obsessively check the five rights three times with each medication administration. Anxiety about making an error should make it impossible to not check. None of us can be perfect, but this redundant and habitual system is proven to reduce errors.

The five rights and the three checks are just the beginning. We'll touch more on patient safety in Chapters 22 and 23.

## References

"In Hospital Deaths from Medical Errors at 195,000 per Year USA." Medical News Today. Available at *www.medicalnewstoday.com/articles/11856.php*. Accessed November 11, 2007.

"Medication Errors Injure 1.5 million People and Cost Billions of Dollars Annually." The National Academies. Available at *www8.nationalacademies.org/onpinews/newsitem.aspx?RecordID=11623*. Accessed January 3, 2008.

# Chapter 8

# Pharmacokinetics: What's the first-pass effect, anyway?

It's time for us to look at how drugs enter our patients, roam to where they are needed, become metabolized, and ultimately leave the body. Let's take this very complex topic and reduce it to four steps to create a framework for our discussion. We will consider absorption, distribution, metabolism, and excretion in sequence. But note that all of these steps could be simultaneous events when someone is taking a regularly scheduled medication.

## All about absorption

We are going to define absorption as the process of drugs moving from the site of administration into the blood (Lehne, Merck). This process entails medications moving across or through cell membranes via:

- Channels or pores: not a common method; usually an option only for very small substances such as electrolytes

- Transport systems: can be passive or require energy (active)

  - Each system moves specific substances

  - Systems can move drugs in or out of a cell

- Direct penetration of the membrane: method used by most drugs

  - Since cell membranes have a lipid layer, direct penetration requires drugs to be lipid soluble

  - Polar molecules (substances having a relative positive and negative pole despite being electrically neutral as a whole) cannot penetrate membranes

  - Ions, or charged particles, cannot penetrate cell membranes

Pharmaceutical companies can "build" medications in such a fashion to affect absorption. Oral medications can be formulated to enhance or slow dissolution and absorption. For example, the type of inactive ingredients and how tightly compressed a tablet is determines how quickly it dissolves. Drugs can also be packaged as capsules with gelatin shells. Capsules filled with liquids tend to have quicker absorption times than those containing powders. Time-released medications can be made by mixing portions of the drug formulated with various dissolution rates. How cool is that?

**Tip:** Here's a critical thinking question: What drug route has immediate, 100% absorption? Exactly! I can see you thinking. Intravenous administration meets the criteria since it is directly injected into the blood. That is why IV drugs have such a quick response.

### A bit about bioavailability

There is a related term we should briefly consider here: bioavailability. This refers to how quickly (and how much) medication reaches the desired target. You will see this term in drug guides and package inserts. It's plain to see that increased absorption rates increases bioavailability.

**Did you know:** Bioavailability is calculated by comparing the amount of PO absorption to IV absorption. The speed of absorption can be important clinically by affecting onset of action, but it does not increase bioavailability. If a drug is 50% bioavailable, a faster absorption rate will not increase the total bioavailability, but simply decrease the time to reaching the 50% bioavailability.

Absorption and bioavailability are affected by patient characteristics in addition to how drugs are formulated. For example, a person who took a couple of aspirin for a headache may notice a delayed effect if the drug was taken after a Burger King Double Whopper® meal. Surprisingly, there are some medications that may actually have increased absorption after a fatty meal. Absorption can also be altered by things such as aging, gastrointestinal disease, and other medications.

## Dipping into distribution

Medical providers (pharmacists, physicians, and nurses) define distribution as the movement of a drug from the blood to the various tissues in the body (Merck, Distribution). This is a pretty straightforward process for commonly used medications:

- The drug is carried to wherever blood flows

- Drugs leave the bloodstream and enter the tissues

  - Some leave the bloodstream slowly or to a lesser extent because they cling to proteins such as albumin found in the blood. These are referred to as protein-bound.

  - Water soluble drugs leave the blood slower, in general, than fat-soluble drugs. They also accumulate in the fluid portions of the body.

  - Lipid (fat) soluble medications leave the blood and accumulate in fatty tissues.

Distribution can be altered by conditions or disease states that alter blood flow (either increase or decrease). For example, a person with vascular changes from diabetes taking an antibiotic for a foot infection may show delayed or absent medication effect because of impaired blood circulation to the extremities. Malnourished persons may show decreased protein binding, resulting in an increase in the drug that reaches the tissues. Also, grossly overweight people may show altered effects with fat-soluble drugs.

## Moving to metabolism

If I need surgery, I want the medications administered by the certified registered nurse anesthetist to render me unconscious and utterly unaware for the planned assault on my body. However, I do not want to remain unconscious indefinitely. We don't want drugs to last forever. Metabolism is one of the processes that accomplishes that for us.

All drugs pass through the liver because all blood flows through hepatic (liver) vessels. While some metabolism takes place in the gastrointestinal tract, bloodstream, or lungs, most of medication metabolism takes place by particular enzymatic pathways in the liver. The liver's chief system responsible for drug metabolism is the cytochrome P-450 enzymatic pathway (CYP450 or CYP). It is important to note that drug metabolism doesn't always result the way one would surmise; it is possible for the liver to metabolize one substance into a more toxic substance. This can happen with acetaminophen, the active ingredient in Tylenol and other nonaspirin pain relievers. When the primary metabolism route is saturated, the secondary metabolic route produces a toxic metabolite.

The most common reason for liver transplants in the United States is biliary atresia (a congenital defect in children), but the number two reason is liver failure from acetaminophen overdose (Emedicine). The liver can alter a drug to enhance excretion by the kidneys, increase the effect (as in the conversion by our liver of codeine to morphine), or activate a pro-drug form to an activated form (Lehne).

Metabolism pathways can be overwhelmed, or saturated, in patients receiving too many medications that rely on hepatic metabolism. Age is also an important factor since the metabolic pathways are not fully operational at birth, become most rapid during late childhood, settle to adult levels during adolescence, and tend to wane in efficiency with age. Alcoholic beverage consumption can slow metabolism. Heavy alcohol consumption with resultant liver damage can permanently impair drug metabolism.

 **Tip:** Consequently, the astute nurse will recognize that the very young and the very old, those taking multiple medications, and heavy alcohol users may need dose modifications (amounts and frequency) in order to avoid toxicity. On the other hand, children may actually need more of a given drug due to their accelerated hepatic metabolism.

## Ending with excretion

Anybody in the class amazed at how fast garbage piles up around at home? How can any small cluster of people manage to fill a large bin and, with similar unstinting aid from neighbors, support a business that sends out a fleet of trucks every week to take these dregs away?

Now, reframe that perspective to examine pharmaceutical consumption. Take a minute to consider how many vitamins, cold pills, and headache tablets you've taken in your life. Add prescription drugs to that image and then include any lotion, anti-itch ointment, or topical analgesic (pain relieving) cream you've used. We're talking tons here! Excretion, the body's refuse service, carried the stuff away.

The kidneys are the most important organ of excretion. We do get rid of some things through our lungs, which is why alcohol shows up on a breathalyzer machine. And some drugs leave in our sweat or other body fluids. For example, the antituberculosis medicine rifampin colors sweat, tears, and urine red (in fact, the tears can permanently stain soft contact lenses). Ions (positively or negatively charged substances), polar molecules (substances with relatively negative and positive ends despite an overall neutral charge), and substances not bound to proteins are all efficiently excreted by the kidneys.

The effectiveness and efficiency of renal excretion can be modified. Excretion can be modulated by altering urine pH. Making the urine more acidic promotes the excretion of weak bases. Alkalinization of urine promotes the excretion of weak acids. It is important to note that aging decreases kidney efficiency, too. At age 80, drug clearance through the kidneys is typically only half what it was at age 30 (Merck, Excretion).

## Some final considerations

We need to reflect on a few last concepts before we finish this pharmacokinetics lesson. To round out our understanding, we need to examine the first-pass effect, the idea of half-life, and the need for adequate blood levels.

### First, the first-pass effect
Our bodies are astonishingly well designed! Consider this: As the digested particles of substances we consume cross intestinal membranes, they are absorbed into our bloodstream. No mystery there, but here is the cool part: The blood flows directly from the gastrointestinal tract to the liver where vigilant defenses come into play. Microbial life forms and foreign proteins are attacked by our immune system, and potentially life-threatening compounds are neutralized by metabolic pathways before they can enter the systemic circulation and poison us.

                               **51**

The downside to this remarkable defense mechanism is known as the first-pass effect. In a cool bit of design, all of this blood first travels to the liver by the portal (doorway) circulation where harmful substances or disease-causing organisms can be removed. Unfortunately, this first-pass effect can markedly reduce the amount of drug in the blood exiting the liver. So, healthcare providers have had to find ways to circumvent these natural defenses. Drugs administered sublingually (under the tongue), such as nitroglycerin for cardiac-associated chest pain, or intravenously, are examples.

**Tip:** You need to consider the first-pass effect when administering drugs that are affected by it. The doses must be higher to make sure enough escapes metabolism, or the medication needs to be given by a route other than oral.

### A full view of half-life

Tabers (2001) defines half-life as the time required by the body to metabolize or inactivate half the amount of a substance. By knowing the half-life of a given medication, it is possible to predict when the effects will wear off. For example, Nitrostat® given sublingually for cardiac-related chest pain begins to work exceedingly fast, but it has a half-life of one to three minutes (Epocrates). Amiodarone, given to treat abnormal heart rhythms, has a half-life of 58 days (Epocrates).

Each medication has a half-life based on how rapidly it is metabolized given its chemical structure. It is important to remember that any factor that alters metabolism or excretion affects (enhances or slows) half-life. Because of this, the half-life for a given drug may vary considerably from patient to patient.

**Tip:** The take-home lessons here are:

- Drugs with a short half-life need to be administered more often and those with a long half-life can be given less often

- Drugs with long half-lives can take a long, long, long time to completely clear from the body

### On the level with blood levels

Consider this: If you have a headache, you have a basic understanding that lets you know that one-tenth of an aspirin tablet is probably not going to do much good. You also have an idea that 10 aspirin tablets probably aren't good for you, even though that amount should nail the headache. Let's consider those intuitive conclusions and say we know there needs to be a minimum effective concentration in our blood in order for the drug to work and we need to avoid a toxic concentration. All medications have these minimum and maximum therapeutic levels, the area between which is known as the therapeutic window.

We would also want our blood level to remain in this window for as long as we needed the medication (antihypertensive, antibiotic, analgesic, etc.) effect. If the drug remains within this window, we will say it has reached a plateau (Lehne).

Let's look at just one more key idea—stay with me here, almost done!

What does half-life have to do with drug levels and plateau? An example is in order: Imagine your nurse practitioner gave you a prescription for a made-up drug, say Jubilation, to increase your overall happiness. The dose is 100 mg, and the drug has a half-life of four days. If you take a dose, four days later you have only 50 mg in your blood. After another four days, you have only half of the remainder, or 25 mg, in your blood. Another four days goes by, and now only half of the half, or 12.5 mg, remains. And in another four days, just 6.25 mg is left. So, we can see that it takes about four half-lives for 94% of this drug to exit the body. If we continue to give doses at appropriate intervals instead of letting the drug wear off, it takes four half-lives for a drug to reach plateau, or steady-state level.

 **Don't forget:** It takes four half-lives to reach plateau and four half-lives for the drug to leave the body.

Whew! We've covered a lot today. You need to know how to define absorption, distribution, metabolism, and excretion, and what can affect each. Also, we talked about the first-pass effect, half-life, and blood levels. Most of it is based on common sense, so don't despair. But remember: Our language needs to be precise, so this is definitely a stellar moment when flash cards would be useful. It would also be a great occasion to give a lecture to the dog!

Go ahead, we'll wait. Then, we'll move on to the ways drugs can be given.

## References

"Absorption." The Merck Manuals Online Medical Library. Available at *www.merck.com/mmpe/sec20/ch303/ch303b.html?qt=drug%20absorption&alt=sh*. Accessed November 12, 2007.

"Distribution." The Merck Manuals Online Medical Library. Available at *www.merck.com/mmpe/sec20/ch303/ch303d.html*. Accessed January 3, 2008.

"Epocrates RX Pro." Drug Reference Guide for the PDA. Available at *www.epocrates.com/products/rxpro*. Accessed November 12, 2007.

"Excretion." The Merck Manuals Online Medical Library. Available at *www.merck.com/mmpe/sec20/ch303/ch303f.html*. Accessed January 3, 2008.

Lehne, R. (2006). *Pharmacology for nursing care,* 6th ed. St. Louis Missouri: Saunders.

"Metabolism." The Merck Manuals Online Medical Library. Available at *www.merck.com/mmpe/sec20/ch303/ch303e.html*. Accessed January 3, 2008.

"Rifadin: Warnings and  precautions." Rx List: The Internet Drug Index. Available at *www.rxlist.com/cgi/generic/rifampin_wcp.htm*. Accessed November 18, 2007.

"Toxicity, Acetaminophen." EMedicine from WebMD. Available at *www.emedicine.com/ped/topic7.htm*. Accessed November 18, 2007.

Venes, D. and Thomas, C. (eds) (2001). *Tabers Cylcopedic Medical Dictionary.* Philadelphia: F.A. Davis Company

# Chapter 9

# Picking the right (or wrong) route

As we start this class, let us first come to an agreement about what we won't be covering: We won't be discussing the specific techniques employed to administer medications. That is the sort of lesson best learned on another day with a clinical component in which to practice newly acquired skills under supervision. Today, we'll focus on: How can medications be given, and what are the advantages and disadvantages of each route?

As we learned from our pharmacokinetics lesson, all medications need to be absorbed into the body and distributed to their sites of action. We will take a look at the different routes and how they vary in convenience, required skill, absorption, and distribution.

 **Don't forget:** We are building on prior knowledge. Remember, the five rights and three checks apply to each of these routes. Also, consider what you've learned about absorption and distribution and how it relates to our present discussion.

## Getting to the root of the routes

### Orally speaking
Wouldn't it be great if all medications could be given orally? No mess, no fuss—anyone who can eat could be medicated! Specific advantages of using the oral route include:

- The oral route doesn't require a ton of cognitive effort from the patient; they just put it in their mouth and swallow.

- Because no needles or other intrusive devices are involved, oral administration can be safer.

- It is also a cheaper, more cost-effective way to give drugs. Think about it: The patient doesn't need high-tech drug delivery systems such as infusion pumps, sterile syringes, or highly trained people to administer a tablet. Tablets or oral liquids are also cheaper to produce than injectable medications.

- In addition, there may be an added measure of safety after oral medication administration. If you mistakenly give the wrong drug or dose, you have alternatives. You can give emetics to induce vomiting, suction it out through a tube, or perhaps administer something else to reduce absorption.

However, there are some fairly significant disadvantages:

- Unconscious people can't swallow. Don't ever test that hypothesis; it's been proven!

- Drug dissolution and absorption can be variable or incomplete due to factors such as stomach contents, gastric pH, gastric motility (how fast the stomach propels its contents into the small intestine), intestinal motility, and so on.

- Some medications, such as insulin or heparin, are destroyed in the stomach, while others such as mannitol cannot be absorbed into the bloodstream.

### Would you prefer parenteral?

Parenteral is actually a cluster of routes rather than a single method. It is derived from Greek words meaning "beside" (para) "intestine" (enteron). Let's take a look at a few of the parenteral routes:

- **Subcutaneous** (SC or SQ, "under the skin"). It is possible to deposit medications just beneath the skin where they are slowly absorbed and enter the bloodstream. This is a common method to administer many drugs including insulin (to treat diabetes) and heparin (to inhibit blood clotting). It has some great advantages, including:

- Not a whole lot of skill is required even though it does involve injecting through a needle. The preferred needles are exquisitely thin (25 gauge, or approximately 0.5 mm) and short (5/8 inch or shorter) (Evans-Smith). So, if you avoid areas close to eyeballs, for example, you are not apt to hit anything vital since we all (excluding people with malnutrition or emaciation) have at least a half inch of fatty tissue beneath the skin. Common subcutaneous sites are the backs of the upper arms, the abdomen, and anterior surfaces of the thighs.

- The equipment involved is not very expensive since these subcutaneous syringes are simple and mass-produced. People with diabetes who need to inject insulin daily (we will talk about that in a future lesson) can purchase 100 disposable syringes for $10–$15 in most pharmacies.

- It provides a way to administer medications that cannot be given orally.

- The patient doesn't need to be awake—or even cooperative—for administration to occur.

However, like the oral route, there are some disadvantages to the subcutaneous approach:

- Generally, this method is suitable for only small dose volumes (1 mL or less) of medication, although larger amounts of fluid are sometimes administered under specific circumstances.

- The needle used breaches the body's defenses and can be a port through which infection can enter.

- Some skill is needed to select appropriate locations and give medications safely. Not all patients or family members can be successfully taught.

- Subcutaneous administration can be uncomfortable.

- Absorption can be slow or variable.

**Intramuscular (IM, "into muscle").** This is a common method to give larger volumes (up to 3–5 mL) when quicker absorption is desired. Some advantages include:

- It is quicker and more reliable absorption than subcutaneous administration

- It can be employed with unresponsive or uncooperative patients

- It is useful to administer medications unable to be administered orally

Again, there are also some disadvantages:

- There is a greater possibility of discomfort (needles are typically 22–20 gauge, or 0.7–0.9 mm, and 1.5-2 inches long)

- There are limited appropriate injection sites

- There are volume limitations

- Some drugs are too irritating to tissues to be administered IM

- A higher degree of skill is needed to safely administer medication

- There is a greater risk of infection

- There is a risk of damage to tissues near injection site (nerves, blood vessels, the muscle itself)

**Intravenous (IV, "into a vein").** This is a commonly used approach seen every day in acute-care nursing practice. There are enormous advantages to this method:

- There is the ability to administer large or small volumes.

- There is the ability to administer substances irritating to tissues in other approaches.

- It is 100% absorption guaranteed! (Remember, absorption by definition is movement of the drug into the bloodstream.)

- It is convenient once a line is inserted.

- It is comfortable (at least more so than IM or SC) once access is achieved.

Some disadvantages include:

- There is significant infection risk. (In fact, it is one of the most common ways in which people become infected while in the hospital.)

- There is significant injury risk. It requires considerable skill to insert and maintain IVs.

- It is generally not for long-term use. There are specific exceptions, including nutrition or chronic medication needs.

- It is uncomfortable to achieve access.

- **Intradermal (ID, "into the skin").** If you have ever had a tuberculosis skin test, you had an intradermal injection. The desired goal here is to instill the medication into the skin—no small task—but not too deep and not too superficial. This method has limited usefulness and requires significant skill.

## Don't forget to consider . . .

There are many possible ways to administer medications for specific purposes (intra-articular into a joint, intraocular into an eyeball, intrathecal into the spinal canal, vaginal, etc.), but we will briefly discuss only a few more common techniques:

- **Rectal** (PR – inserted into the rectum). One method that is typically forgotten in medication administration discussions among nursing students is the rectal route. Antiemetics (vomiting preventers), anxyiolytics (anxiety relievers), analgesics (pain relievers), and others can all be administered rectally. Relatively little training is required, and this approach can be used in people with diminished alertness.

 **Don't forget:** When using the rectal route, absorption is variable, particularly if the medication is expelled.

- **Topical.** Many medications can now be administered as creams or patches applied to the skin surface. These include hormone replacement preparations, antihypertensives to lower blood pressure, vasodilators to reduce cardiac workload, potent analgesics to treat cancer pain, and nicotine to ease the pangs of smoking cessation. What a cool idea! They can be used by patients with impaired swallowing, and you can teach any patient or family member how to apply them.

 **Don't forget:** When using the topical route, absorption is variable and discarded patches can be extremely hazardous to others, particularly children and pets.

- **Optic and otic routes.** These are used to medicate eyes and ears, respectively. The brilliant usefulness here is you can apply medications directly where needed without needing to be as concerned with systemic effects on the rest of the body. For example, timolol is used to reduce pressure within the eyeball in persons with glaucoma. It would theoretically work if given orally, but this nonselective beta blocker (we will look at these more closely in another lesson) could unnecessarily drop the blood pressure, slow the heart, and cause wheezing (remember ABBA from Chapter 4; there is no statute of limitations on knowledge!).

**Let's sum up this lesson:**
We've learned that drugs can be administered by different routes to accommodate various medication and patient needs. There are advantages and disadvantages to each. AND the five rights and three checks ALWAYS APPLY (don't mean to shout, but I get worked up)!

Okay, we've avoided it long enough. We need to dig deep into math now; it'll be okay, trust me!

## References

Evans-Smith, P. (2005). *Taylor's Clinical Nursing Skills*. Philadelphia: Lipponcott, Williams & Wilkins.

Venes, D. and Thomas, C. (eds) (2001). *Taber's Cylcopedic Medical Dictionary*. Philadelphia: F.A. Davis Company.

# Chapter 10

# Put the 'A' in math

Yes, it's true. The time is here. We actually need to talk about math and do some problems!

In this lesson, we are going to refresh and confirm some old knowledge. Then we will try out and solidify some practical application strategies. At the end of this class, you will feel confident with all of the pharmacology math situations you are likely to encounter as a practicing staff nurse. Now, sit down, close your eyes, and take a slow, deep, cleansing breath. Feel your body becoming relaxed and centered. Are you ready? Let's ease into it . . .

## Let's begin with the basics

We need to begin by going back to elementary school. We will actually use fractions, ratios, and proportions to solve commonly occurring calculations. Remember the fraction rules:

- In 1/4, 1 is the numerator and 4 is the denominator.

- If you wish to add 1/2 + 2/3, recall that you need a common denominator. In this case, the common denominator is 6 (found by multiplying the denominators, 2 x 3).

- If you wish to add 1 1/2 + 2 1/4, remember you need to convert to improper fractions = 3/2 + 9/4, then find the common denominator 6/4 + 9/4 = 15/4 or 3 3/4 .

- You also need a common denominator when you subtract one fraction from another. Is it starting to come back to you? Good!

- If you wanted to multiply 5/6 x 2/5, remember, you just multiply the numerators and denominators straight across and then reduce to lowest terms: 5/6 x 2/5 = 10/30 = 1/3.

- When dividing fractions such as 3/4 ÷ 4/5, you invert the second fraction and multiply: 3/4 x 5/4 = 15/16.

**Tip:** This is a good time to talk about reducing to lowest terms. Remember that 12/20 can be reduced to 3/5. Look to see if the two numbers share common factors, such as 2, 3, or 5, and then divide both numerator and denominator by the factor.

- Fractions can be used as ratios and proportions to solve problems. For example: 3/4 = X/12. We cross multiply and find that 4X = 36, X=9

## Don't fear the decimal

Why don't we do a quick review of decimals? Look at this example: "0.12345." Note a couple of things. First, we are ALWAYS going to use a leading zero to the left of the decimal point and will NEVER write the number as ".12345." (Sorry for shouting.) The reason is safety. If someone overlooks the decimal, they may mistake the number for "12,345!"

Secondly, let's recall the decimal places. So in our illustration, 1 is in the tenths place, 2 is in the hundredths, 3 is in the thousandths, etc. The only real tricky thing we need to review about decimals is relative sizes.

### Look at the following numbers:
A. 0.012       B. 0.0122       C. 0.01221       D. 0.0123

Which is the smallest decimal? No, not quite right; someone raised their hand and said "C," which kind of reflexively makes sense since it "goes out" farthest from the decimal. Can you see, though, that it is really a whopping 1/100,000 bigger than "B"? "A" is the smallest, as it has a zero in the ten-thousandths place.

Take a deep breath; just two more things to review!

Percent just describes a ratio in terms of something per 100. Ten percent means 10 out of every 100, 20% = 20 out of 100, and so on. A 10% solution in medicine or chemistry means 10 grams of solute (the medicine or substance you are interested in) in 100 milliliters of solvent (solution used to dissolve the solute, often water). Officially, it is always grams (g) per milliliter (mL). If I were to ask how many grams of medicine are in 300 mL of a 10% solution, can you see that 10% means 10 g out of every 100 mL? Let's set up a ratio: $10/100 = X/300 \rightarrow 100 X = 3000$ or $X = 30$ g.

## The great thing about estimating

**Tip:** Estimate before you solve any medication math problem.

The great thing about estimating is that this little reflective pause to consider the nuances of the problem will immediately let you know if you inadvertently wander off in the wrong direction. Need an example? Here you go: The doctor orders Amoxicillin 250 mg every six hours. It comes in 500 mg tablets. You should give _____ tablets per dose.

There are a few numbers here. You need to give 250 mg. The tablets each contain 500 mg. There's something about six hours. Let's estimate. First, determine that the patient will get a dose every six hours. Since it is the same dose every six hours, you don't need to care about the six. Great, one number gone! Is 250 mg bigger or smaller than 500 mg? I heard someone shout out "smaller." Absolutely! So it's safe to estimate that since you need to give 250 mg, you will give something smaller than one tablet. That's as far as we are going to go. Estimates are just that, trying to find the general direction and relative amounts.

Now, if in your attempts to solve the problem, you come up with the answer "two" because you mistakenly divide 500 mg by 250 mg, you immediately know that is wrong. Whenever you need to solve a problem, the first step is to read it s-l-o-w-l-y and c-a-r-e-f-u-l-l-y. The second is to estimate. The third step is to crank up the dimensional analysis machine.

## Dealing with dimensional analysis

Even the name sounds painful! Dimensional analysis, also known as the way to true pharmacological math happiness and pure contentment, is a method of approaching problems that begins with something you know that is changed into what you want to know through a series of conversions.

The conversions are written as fractions. Remember how we learned previously that there are 5 mL in a teaspoon? We will write that as 5mL/1tsp or 1tsp/5ml. This method relies on all the principles we have considered in this lesson so far. Why don't we look at the problem we examined earlier?

The doctor orders Amoxicillin 250 mg every six hours. It comes in 500 mg tablets. You should give _____ tablets per dose.

**Here's what we know:**

- Need to give 250 mg, written as 250mg/dose or 1dose/250mg

- Gets one dose every six hours or four doses per day, can be written as 4doses/1day or 1day/4doses

- 500 mg tablets, written as 500mg/1tab or 1tab/500mg

**Here's what we want to find out:**
- How many tablets per dose

**Here's what we do:**

1. X tabs/dose [this is what we want to find out] =?

2. What do we put on the right side of the equal sign? Do we know anything about tabs? Sure, 1 tab = 500 mg, and we can write it as a ratio or fraction: 1tab/500mg or 500mg/1tab. We want tabs in the numerator (left side of the = sign) so we will choose the first method of writing it. So now we have:

3. X tabs/dose = 1tab/500mg

4. Now we have mg in the denominator on the right, so our equation really is not equal yet. Can we multiply by another conversion to get rid of mg? How about:

5. X tabs/dose = 1tab/500mg x 250mg/1dose

6. We know from algebra that if we have something in the numerator and denominator, we can "cancel" them. So in this case, mg is in the denominator of the first factor and the numerator in the second, so we can cancel them. When we multiply everything out, we have:

7. X tabs/dose = 1tab/500 x 250/1dose = 250tabs/500dose = 0.5 tabs/dose

Isn't that cool? Of course, this problem is so simple you could do it in your head. The method also points out what we don't need to know; you can see we didn't use the second bulleted information because we didn't need to! Why don't we try it with something just a touch more complex?

Your patient is on a heparin drip. A 250 mL bag of D5W contains 25,000 units of heparin. Your patient needs to receive 1500 units per hour. How many mL/hr should you run the IV at?

**Here's what we know:**

- 250mL/25,000 units

- 1500 units/hr

**The solution:** Xml/hr = 250mL/25000 units x 1500 units/hr = 15mL/hr

## Practice makes perfect!

Here are a bunch of problems for you. Answers follow, but don't look at them until you solve the problem. Some of you might still take a peek. The answers will make sense, so these souls will erroneously claim, "I know how to do these!" as they move on to the next lesson. Don't be one of them.

1. The order reads "Lanoxin®, 0.125 mg IVP every a.m." Lanoxin® comes in a vial labeled 0.5 mg per mL. You should give _____mL.

2. You are to give NS at a rate of 30 mL/hour. Your tubing is mini-drip tubing with a drop factor of 60 (60 drops per mL). How many drops/minute do you set the IV at?

3. The doctor orders Cytoxan® 375 mg in 500 mL D5W to be given over two hours. You are running it on a pump. How many mL per hour do you give?

4. The doctor's order reads to give metoprolol 200 mg four times a day. You have 100 mg tablets available. How many tablets do you administer with each dose?

5. The doctor's order reads to give metoprolol 200 mg four times a day. You have 100 mg tablets available. How many total mg does the patient receive each day?

6. You are to infuse 1000 mL D5W over eight hours. How many mL/hour do you administer?

7. You are to administer ganciclovir 5 mg/kg IV in 100 mL of NS over one hour. Your patient weighs 75 kg. How many mL/hour do you administer?

8. Your patient is to receive aminophylline 2 grams in 1000mL D5W. It is to infuse at a rate of 0.5 mg/kg/hour, and your patient weighs 65 kg. How many mL/hour do you set the pump at?

9. Your patient is on a dobutamine drip, and it is to run at 10mcg/kg/min. Your patient weighs 165 lbs. You have 750 mg of dobutamine in 250 mL D5W. How many mL/hour do you set the IV to run at?

10. **Extra credit question:** A child weighs 55 lbs. What would be the daily maintenance fluid intake this child should have? (Remember: For the first 10 kg, the child needs 100mL /kg, for the second 10 kg, the child should receive 50mL/kg, and for each kg above 20 kg, the child should receive another 20mL/kg).

**Answers**

1. The order reads "Lanoxin®, 0.125 mg IVP every a.m.." Lanoxin® comes in a vial labeled 0.5 mg per mL. You should give _____ mL.

   *X ml = 0.125mg x 1ml/0.5mg = 0.25 mL*

2. You are to give NS at a rate of 30mL/hour. Your tubing is mini-drip tubing with a drop factor of 60. How many drops/minute do you set the IV at?

   *x gtts(drops)/min = 30mL/hr x 1hr/60 min x 60gtts/1 mL = 30 gtts/min*

3. The doctor orders Cytoxan® 375 mg in 500 mL D5W to be given over two hours. You are running it on a pump. How many mL per hour do you give?

   *X mL/hr = 500mL/2 hrs = 250mL/hr*

4. The doctor's order reads to give metoprolol 200 mg four times a day. You have 100 mg tablets available. How many tablets do you administer with each dose?

   *X tabs/dose = 200mg/dose x 1tab/100mg = 2 tabs*

5. The doctor's order reads to give metoprolol 200 mg four times a day. You have 100 mg tablets available. How many total mg does the patient receive each day?

   *X mg/day = 200mg/dose x 4doses/day = 800 mg*

6. You are to infuse 1000 mL D5W over eight hours. How many mL/hour do you administer?

   *X mL/hr = 1000mL/8hr = 125mL/hr*

7. You are to administer ganciclovir 5mg/kg IV in 100 mL of NS over one hour. Your patient weighs 75 kg. How many mL/hour do you administer?

   *100mL/hr*

8. Your patient is to receive aminophylline 2 grams in 1000 mL D5W. It is to infuse at a rate of 0.5mg/kg/hour, and your patient weighs 65 kg. How many mL/hour do you set the pump at?

   *x mL/hr = 0.5mg/kghr x 65 kg/1 x 1g/1000 mg x 1000mL/2 g = 16.25 mL/hr*

9. Your patient is on a dobutamine drip, and it is to run at 10mcg/kg/min. Your patient weighs 165 lbs. You have 750 mg of dobutamine in 250 mL D5W. How many mL/hour do you set the IV to run at?

   *X mL/hr = 10mcg/kgmin x 1kg/2.2 lbs x 165lbs/1 x 1mg/1000 mcg x 60min/1hr x 250cc/750mg = 15  mL/hr*

10. **Extra credit question:** A child weighs 55 lbs. What would be the daily maintenance fluid intake this child should have? (Remember: For the first 10 kg, the child needs 100mL/kg, for the second 10 kg, the child should receive 50mL/kg, and for each kg above 20 kg, the child should receive another 20mL/kg).

    *X kg = 55 lbs x 1kg/2.2 lbs = 25 kg.*

    *For first 10 kg = 10 kg x 100mL/kg = 1000 mL.*

    *For second 10 kg = 10 kg x 50mL/kg = 500 mL.*

    *For remainder, 5 kg x 20mL/kg = 100 mL.*

    *Adding them = 1000 mL + 500 mL + 100 mL = 1600 mL*

# Chapter 11

# How do drugs work?

Welcome back. The lesson for today will focus on how drugs actually work. This is going to be one of the shorter chapters. (Okay, enough clapping already!) Despite the brevity, every concept is gold. And the really brilliant part? The content is not too difficult and really makes intuitive sense. Devote some time and reflection to today's class because it lays the foundation for understanding many of our subsequent topics.

## Receptors and reactions

**Tip:** The key concept here is that drugs either act on receptors or act in chemical or mechanical reactions.

Some examples might be in order at this point: Think back to your anatomy and physiology classes. Do you recall that there are neurons (nerve cells) innervating the heart? These nerve cells provide competing stimuli. Some speed up the heart (sympathetic) and some slow it down (parasympathetic) when their respective receptors are stimulated or blocked. Cardiac medications, for example, stimulate or inhibit those receptors. (We'll touch more on receptors later.)

We also said medications can act in chemical reactions. Strictly speaking, receptor activity relies on complex chemical reactions. But at the moment, we are looking at something much more basic. The clearest example might be the weak bases we swallow to neutralize stomach acid when we have heartburn. Imagine yourself cramming for an exam (not that you do that) and consuming copious amounts of coffee in an effort to remain awake and alert. The slow burn sets in . . . and your stomach needs something and it needs to come quickly. Picture yourself taking your favorite antacid and obtaining comfort. It is a simple chemical reaction of a weak base soaking up excess hydrogen ions from acid and blunting the effects of other irritants in the beverage. Ah, relief.

Finally, there are medications that act mechanically. Bulk-forming laxatives illustrate this quite nicely. Patients sometimes develop constipation. We need to be clear what we mean, though: difficulty in passing stool or incomplete/ infrequent hard stools (Mosby). It would be inappropriate and potentially harmful to administer laxatives solely because a patient thought he should have a bowel movement every day. Anyway, one treatment is to administer insoluble fiber products that cannot be absorbed into the body from the gas-trointestinal tract. These products, when taken with sufficient water, do nothing but add bulk to the stool. They enlarge and soften the stool, which eases its passage through the colon.

## The trick to understanding receptors

Let's first talk about receptors in more detail. Picture yourself in a rush trying to get to class or work on time. You are running late but need the caffeine fix, so you pull into a drive-through and fling them a couple of bills in exchange for a skim latte with an extra shot of espresso. You tip the cardboard cup back for a hefty swig. The coffee is unexpectedly hot, and you reflexively move it swiftly away from your mouth to shield yourself from a bad burn. There are sensory and motor nerves involved here, but let's focus on just the extensor muscle group in the dorsal surface of your hand and forearm that pulled the cup away.

Imagine that the lower motor neuron from your spinal cord is directly attached to that group. Thus, the nerve would endlessly communicate with that muscle. Since that extensor group of muscles can only extend, your hand would perpetually be pulled back—or at least until your muscles totally fatigued. In reality, there is a little gap, the synaptic cleft, between the end of the nerve and the muscle. These gaps exist between one nerve and another— the presynaptic and postsynaptic neurons. A neurotransmitter chemical released from the presynaptic neuron floats across that gap and carries the nerve impulse to the postsynaptic neuron when muscular action is needed. The presence or absence of the chemical determines whether or not impulses are transmitted and allows a wide functional range of activity. This allows that extensor group of muscles to extend or not extend.

 **Don't forget:** Many medications exert a powerful effect by enhancing or inhibiting neurotransmitters.

There are many known (and unknown but postulated) neurotransmitting substances. Common neurotransmitters include:

- Acetylcholine

- Epinephrine

- Norepinephrine

- Gamma aminobutyric acid (GABA)

- Dopamine

- Serotonin

There are different transmitters for various tissues and parts of body systems, which is an incredible piece of design. Consider this: What would it be like if the same type of neurotransmitter-receptor system your body uses to cause nasal drainage in response to irritation was used to regulate heart rate? The allergy pill you might take to dry up your drippy nose might also slow or stop your heart. Multiple types of receptors actuated by many unique neurotransmitters are definitely a stunning idea!

 **Tip:** Here's one of the key points of our discussion: These neurotransmitters are made, stored, released, gathered in again (reuptake is the technical term for this gathering), and metabolized (Porth). Medications directed at receptors can affect only those five processes. Drugs cannot stimulate a receptor to produce entirely new actions or responses; they can stimulate, accentuate, diminish, or totally prevent only that receptor's current action (Lehne).

 **Don't forget:**
All medications that inhibit or promote receptor function work by:

- Affecting neurotransmitter production

- Altering neurotransmitter storage

- Regulating neurotransmitter (release)

- Influencing the amount of time the neurotransmitter remains in the synaptic gap

- Speeding up or slowing down neurotransmitter metabolism

Knowing how medications affect receptors will also allow you to accurately predict (and prepare your patients for) likely side effects. Parts of the body that share similar receptors can all respond to a particular medication.

## Ugh! Chemistry and physics again?

As we stated above, some medications produce effects without stimulating or inhibiting receptors. Here are some examples:

- We noted earlier that some create a chemical reaction. Magnesium hydroxide, when given in small doses, acts chemically as a weak base or proton acceptor and is effective as an antacid. Hydrogen ions from stomach acids are neutralized, heartburn symptoms diminish, and comfort and good humor are restored (Wilson, et al.). When magnesium hydroxide is given in larger doses, it acts in a different way. It promotes osmotic retention of water within the lumen of the bowel, which, in turn, stimulates peristalsis.

- Sucralfate behaves in a completely different way. It is a complex of aluminum hydroxide and sulfated sucrose used to protect damaged areas of gastric mucosa (Wilson, et al.). Once swallowed, this tablet becomes a paste that adheres to eroded or ulcerated areas in the stomach where it absorbs bile, blocks the enzyme pepsin, and guards the stomach lining against damage from gastric acids. It too accomplishes its tasks without stimulating or blocking receptors.

- Mineral oil, on the other hand, has a direct mechanical effect. If someone has constipation and is unable to pass a hard fecal mass, mineral oil is sometimes administered rectally as an enema. The oil lubricates and softens the feces and promotes passage of the stool (Wilson, et al.).

## The rundown on drugs

In summary, we've that seen most drugs act in two ways:

- They affect the neurotransmitter function in the synapses between nerves
- They have direct chemical or mechanical effects

We've determined that there are many neurotransmitters and that all progress through five stages that can be influenced by medications: production, storage, release, reuptake, and metabolism. Finally, we also examined how some medications create effects by acting chemically or mechanically, rather than affecting neurotransmitters.

Whew! A short lesson but one full of important concepts! Let's move on to dangerous interactions and compare old drugs with new medications.

## References

Lehne, R. (2007). *Pharmacology for Nursing Care*, 6th ed. St. Louis: Elsevier.

Myers, T. (ed). (2006). *Mosby's Dictionary of Medicine, Nursing & Health Professions*, 7th ed. St. Louis: Elsevier.

Porth, C. (2004). *Essentials of Pathophysiology*, 6th ed. Philadelphia: Lippincott Williams & Wilkins.

Wilson, B., Shannon, M., Shields, K. & Stang, C. (2007) *Nurse's Drug Guide 2007*. Upper Saddle River, New Jersey: Prentice Hall.

# Chapter 12

# Let's get intertwined in interactions

We have just a few additional items to study before we start looking at specific medications. This lesson will help us consider the hazards of drug interactions. Haven't we all seen people suffering from a cold take one pill to reduce the runny nose, another couple to extinguish a fever, a tablespoon of syrup to quell a cough, and maybe a multivitamin or extra vitamin C? Some of you may already be seeing patients as nursing students or new graduates and have found that patients frequently take five or 10 medications together several times throughout the day. Have you ever wondered if that is dangerous? Or have you questioned whether the combination inhibited or inactivated any of the individual drugs? We are going to ponder that in this lesson.

Perhaps you also recall the United States National Library of Medicine DailyMed Web site we mentioned in Chapter 1 as an excellent resource for current information on marketed drugs. It now lists information for 3,458 (it listed 3,408 in Chapter 1) medications. There are new medications hitting the market every week, and you have to wonder: Did the old ones quit working? When does a drug become obsolete? Are the new ones better? We'll spend a few moments on that topic, too, in this class. Let's get started!

## Into the interactions we go . . .

Imagine you are a patient with atrial fibrillation, a condition in which the atria (upper chambers in the heart) merely quiver and no longer contribute to the heart's pumping action. Your ventricles don't quite know how to respond, so they attempt to keep up. Your heart rate is irregular and thumping along at 140 beats a minute as you lie quietly in bed hoping this will all just go away. Cardiac output decreases and blood turbulently swirling in the atria puts you at risk for blood clot development (Porth). Your physicians have tried multiple medications without lasting success, and then the cardiologist brings out the big gun: amiodarone. After just a couple of doses, your heart begins to behave itself. Your cardiac output improves, the relentless and frightening palpitations in the center of your chest cease, and you are back to normal. There is just one catch: Your nurse gives you a long list of medicines that may dangerously interact with amiodarone.

### And amiodarone interacts with . . .

The list of medications that interact with amiodarone includes: cisapride, dofetilide, phenothiazines, pimozide, protease inhibitors, quinolones, anastozole, azithromycin, azole antifungals, bile binding resins, ciprofloxacin, clarithromycins, clozapine, codeine, COX2 inhibitors, digoxin, duloxetine, eplerenone, ergotamine, isoniazid, montelukast, quetiapine, quinidine . . . and another 50 or so medications or drug classes (Epocrates). The drugs listed above illustrate a wide spectrum. Some of them treat heart arrhythmias or abnormal heart beat patterns, (digoxin, quinidine, dofetilide), but others are common antibiotics (azithromycin, ciprofloxacin) or antibiotic classes (quinolones). Isoniazid treats tuberculosis, while quetiapine and clozapine are important antipsychotics.

**Watch out:** When most of these drugs are taken by a person also taking amiodarone, the person is at an increased risk for fatal heart arrhythmias or altered drug levels due to competition with a hepatic (liver) metabolic pathway.

Remember our discussion about pharmacokinetics? We looked at metabolism, including the CYP450 system responsible for many of the amiodarone drug interactions.

**Don't forget:** There is no statute of limitations on knowledge. You'll ace pharmacology and other courses by regularly reviewing prior content. Earlier information often is the substrate for current topics, and giving the brain a booster shot by looking at old lessons improves current academic performance!

Here's the next layer of information: When drugs are metabolized by the liver, the metabolites or end products are often physiologically active too! That is true with amiodarone—it has a metabolite that is active (Epocrates).

 **Tip:** Here's the deal: If you are taking two medications, your physician or nurse practitioner can reasonably predict what will happen in the majority of cases. If you are taking three, four, five, or more drugs, all bets are off.

Trying to predict interactions between the drugs and their metabolites and the metabolites of the metabolites becomes an exercise in wizardry. There are some helpful computer programs available these days that look for common or dangerous interactions, but like all creations, they are imperfect.

## Let's go over the counter and outside the box

Remember, we learned in an earlier chapter that any substance that had desired pharmacologic effects has potential adverse effects. Two aspirin might be good for a headache, but 50 may be harmful. Two aspirin and two ibuprofen tablets may also be harmful. Aspirin and ibuprofen (brand names include Motrin® and Advil®) both belong to the nonsteroidal anti-inflammatory drug (NSAID) class.

 **Tip:** Taking two members of the same class increases the risk of adverse effects.

Let's also consider a different perspective. If you look at the label of a generic bottle of aspirin, you will find a warning about potential gastric irritation and bleeding. Ginkgo biloba, an herbal remedy taken to improve memory and promote clear thinking, also has anticoagulant properties. When it is taken by people also using prescribed anticoagulants, there is an enhanced risk of bleeding and hemorrhagic stroke (Lehne).

 **Tip:** The message here is we need to be just as concerned about interactions with "safe" OTC meds and "natural" remedies.

## Finding out about food

Have you looked at the label on a bottle of generic aspirin lately? A quick glance at a typical label reveals that "if you consume three or more alcoholic drinks every day, ask your doctor whether you should take aspirin or other pain/fever reducers." The combination of the two can precipitate extreme gastric bleeding.

Of course, that's just one example. What about other foods? How about grapefruit juice?

Interactions between grapefruit juice and medications became a hot issue in the late 1980s. Researchers learned that it contains natural substances that can affect the way certain prescription medications are metabolized by a particular enzyme named CYP3A4 (Center for Food Drug Interaction, Research, and Education). Competition for this metabolic pathway permits reduced metabolism and a prolonged effect of the drug in persons who consume grapefruit juice.

There are many foods that interact with medications. The effect of warfarin (an anticoagulant prescribed to inhibit abnormal blood clot formation) is inhibited by foods containing its antidote: vitamin K.

**Click:** Now might be a good time for a homework assignment. Google "vitamin K rich foods," and see what you get. I had 2,370,000 hits in 0.27 seconds.

## So how do I keep my patients safe?

What is the final word regarding interactions? Your patient may be taking multiple medications. Each of those medications could have active metabolites that interact with the other drugs and their metabolites. Your patient may also be eating a wide range of foods, taking a few over-the-counter medications, and supplementing with alternative remedies.

What is going to happen?

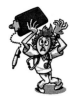

**Don't panic:** The solid truth is no one knows with any degree of certainty. We need to have a plan to minimize the risk. Here it is:

1.  Anytime you start a patient on a new medication—or stop a current medication—you need to carefully scrutinize his or her list of current meds to look for potential interactions. As a nurse, you share this responsibility with physicians and pharmacists.

2.  We are always going to urge our patients to forthrightly disclose everything they are taking, and we are going to teach them why.

3.  We are always going to encourage our patients to use a single pharmacy where they can establish a professional relationship with the pharmacist, who also will vigilantly monitor interaction risk with prescribed and OTC medications using computerized drug information databases.

## Old drugs vs. new drugs: Which is better?

Now let's move on to the second topic of today: all the new drugs hitting the market. Pharmaceutical companies can patent drugs for 20 years. A company has exclusive rights to produce the drug (and charge whatever the market will tolerate) as soon as the drug is approved and for the remaining length of the patent. The federal Food and Drug Administration (FDA) regulations state: "Patents can be expired before drug approval, issued after drug approval, and anywhere in between. Exclusivity is granted upon approval of a drug product if the statutory requirements are met. Some drugs have both patent and exclusivity protection while others have just one or none" (FDA). Essentially, this means once a company develops a new medication, the race is on to recoup the cost of development and earn profits before the patent and exclusive rights expire. It is possible to retain exclusivity by first marketing the new drug as the most effective new treatment for whatever ailment it has been approved. Then, when exclusive rights are about to expire, the company can create the "new and improved" version, developing an extended release formulation, for example.

So, are new drugs always better?

They may be more convenient, but new formulations or new members of a particular drug class may be no more effective than currently available medications. This is not to say innovation is ineffective or unwarranted. We will see in our upcoming antimicrobial lesson how ongoing new antibiotic development is critical in protecting us from rapidly evolving virulent bacterial beasties. The lesson is to be aware of the distinction between effectiveness and convenience.

## On topic with 'off-label' drugs

It's time to move on to the last topic of this lesson. Just what exactly is meant by "off-label" use?

The FDA approves medications for a particular use based on extensively reviewed clinical trial data. Although drug companies cannot promote off-label use, once the drug is approved, physicians can exercise professional judgment and prescribe it for any condition. Paroxetine, for example, is a selective serotonin reuptake inhibitor (SSRI) approved for depression, obsessive-compulsive disorder, panic attacks, generalized anxiety disorder, post-traumatic stress disorder, and premenstrual dysphoric disorder. It is used off label for diabetic neuropathy (painful or distressing numbness or sensations from diabetes related nerve damage), migraine headaches, and fibromyalgia among other things. The safety and effectiveness of treating fibromyalgia has not been formally determined by the FDA, but some physicians and nurse practitioners have found paroxetine to provide relief to their patients. Often, these "off-label" uses still have case reports or case series published in the literature by the clinicians who are successfully using them.

One of the more interesting situations involves Wellbutrin® (buproprion), which was first marketed as an antidepressant. Medical providers noticed these depressed people were smoking less, and the drug was prescribed off label as a smoking cessation aid. Zyban® is another brand name for the same substance meant to overcome the stigma of taking a mental health drug for smoking cessation.

Good work, everyone! We've come a long way in these past few chapters. We've looked at the hurdles—real and perceived—that we need to jump over to conquer our study of pharmacology. We've learned the language, developed a firm grasp on medication math, and are gaining a solid understanding of how drugs work for our benefit despite associated risks.

Okay, time to move on to the next level. Let's begin our tour of body systems with neurology and mental health medications . . .

# References

"DailyMed." U.S. National Library of Medicine, National Institutes of Health, Department of Health and Human Services. Available at *http://dailymed.nlm.nih.gov*. Accessed October 21, 2007.

"Epocrates RX Pro." Drug Reference Guide for the PDA. Available at *www.epocrates.com/products/rxpro*. Accessed October 21, 2007.

"Frequently Asked Questions on Patents and Exclusivity." Food and Drug Administration. Available at *www.fda.gov/cder/ob/faqs.htm*. Accessed December 1, 2007.

"Grapefruit Juice general information." Center for Food-Drug Interaction Research and Education, University of Florida. Available at *www.druginteractioncenter.org/profe.php?interaction_category=9*. Accessed December 12, 2007.

Lehne, R. (2007). *Pharmacology for Nursing Care*, 6th ed. St. Louis: Elsevier.

Porth, C. (2004). *Essentials of Pathophysiology*, 6th ed. Philadelphia: Lippincott Williams & Wilkins.

Springhouse. (2003). *Professional Guide to Pathophysiology*. Philadelphia: Lippincott Williams & Wilkins.

# Part Three

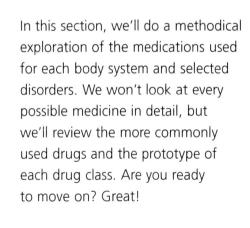

In this section, we'll do a methodical exploration of the medications used for each body system and selected disorders. We won't look at every possible medicine in detail, but we'll review the more commonly used drugs and the prototype of each drug class. Are you ready to move on? Great!

# Chapter 13

# Think about it: Neurological and mental health medications

The nervous system is divided into the central nervous system and the peripheral nervous system. The central nervous system consists of the brain and spinal cord. The remaining peripheral nervous system has voluntary and autonomic (automatic, or without the need for conscious control) components.

One focus of this lesson will be the central nervous system because central nervous system pathology is the root for many familiar disorders. We will also be concerned with the autonomic nervous system since its manipulation by various medications is an important component in treating many diseases ranging from hypertension (elevated blood pressure) to glaucoma (elevated pressure in the eye).

## A trip to the central nervous system

Let's look at the drugs used to treat pain and a couple of common central nervous system diseases as a way to introduce how we will learn medications. Remember to learn the general information common to all the members of a given class first by concentrating on the prototype drug. Then learn the important considerations of particular drugs within the class.

## Facing the pain

There isn't a person in the class who hasn't felt pain. If we took a poll, we would find a wide variety of injuries or disease leading to the sensation. We will learn more about specific over-the-counter medications in Chapter 20, but it seems appropriate to learn about opioid pain relievers that act on the central nervous system in this lesson. Opioid refers to the opium poppy from which the first opioids were derived.

We will look at two kinds of pain:

- Nociception (from tissue injury)

- Neuropathic (from nerve injury)

The first type is what we usually think of—we stub our toe or get a sunburn and experience nociception. Tissue is damaged and sends out a signal along intact nerves letting us know.

Neuropathic pain is different. In this case, the nerve's ability to carry impulses is impaired due to damage. This results in an altered sensation. Have you ever hit your funny bone (ulnar nerve where it travels along the rear of the elbow) and felt the burning and tingling sensation in your middle, ring, and little fingers? The fingers were okay even though they were the things that hurt, and that is neuropathic pain.

Imagine that same sensation in your hand, your foot, or an entire leg. There are people who have horrible neuropathic pain every day due to the effects of crushing type injuries or chronic diseases, such as diabetes. Neuropathic pain is treated using the opioids listed in the table below and some of the seizure medications in later tables.

1. System review: There are three different types of opioid receptors, but all opioids primarily work on mu receptors in the brain. The mu receptors are responsible for pain relief as well as sedation, respiratory depression, euphoria (the high that drug users look for), physical dependence, and slowed gastrointestinal motility. Kappa receptor activation does give some pain relief, sedation, and slowed GI motility, but no euphoria. Delta receptor activation may provide some pain relief as well. Drugs that stimulate receptors are agonists; those that block them are antagonists. Opioids can be agonists at one or more of the receptors and are called pure agonists. Selected medications that can block mu yet stimulate kappa and delta receptors are called agonist-antagonists.

2.  Drug class information:

- General indications: used to treat moderate to severe pain; some used to treat cough.

- General administration routes: can be administered by any route.

- General effects: reduced pain, cough suppression.

- General adverse effects: slowed breathing (respiratory depression), nausea, vomiting, constipation, physical and psychological dependence leading to withdrawal symptoms if medication is stopped abruptly, urinary retention, orthostatic hypotension (blood pressure falls when shifting from lying or sitting position to standing).

- Nursing considerations: give bowel program of laxatives or stool softeners, watch for excessive sedation, monitor respiratory status; antidote is naloxone (Narcan®), which is a strong antagonist at both mu kappa and delta receptors.

**Let's look at some specific medications:**

### Figure 2: Painkillers

| Medication | Specific indications | Potential adverse effects | Nursing considerations |
|---|---|---|---|
| Morphine (prototype) | Moderate to severe pain | Respiratory depression, head injury (raises intracranial pressure) | Bowel program, monitor respirations |
| Hydromorphone (Dilaudid®) | Moderate to severe pain | Respiratory depression | Bowel program, monitor respirations |
| Fentanyl (Duragesic®) | Moderate to severe pain | Respiratory depression; should not be used unless patient accustomed to receiving opioids | Comes as skin patches, oral pills, oral suckers/lozenges |
| Codeine | Mild to moderate pain; very effective cough suppressant | Known particularly for causing nausea and vomiting | Almost always given with nonopioid (such as acetaminophen) to enhance pain relief |
| Oxycodone (Oxycontin®, for example) | Moderate to severe pain | Extended release tablets can cause overdose if crushed or chewed | General considerations apply |
| Hydrocodone (Vicodin® or Lortab® for example) | Moderate to severe pain | Extended release tablets can cause overdose if crushed or chewed | General considerations apply |

### A portrayal of Parkinson's disease

First, let's look at a few numbers to help us put things into perspective. How common are neurological disorders? Let's toss out a question: How many in the class know or are related to someone with Parkinson's disease? Thought so, nearly every one of you has a hand up.

**Did you know:** The National Parkinson Foundation reports 60,000 people are newly diagnosed each year and approximately 1.5 million Americans have the disease (About Parkinson).

The disease was first described in 1817 by James Parkinson. Afflicted persons exhibit symptoms such as rigid muscles, tremor, akinesia (lack of movement), drooling, a mask-like expression, difficulty swallowing and speaking, and orthostatic hypotension (blood pressure plummets when patient rises from lying or sitting position). We will look at some of the medications used to treat Parkinson's because the disease is so common. It is important to keep in mind that the disease worsens with time and that all medications eventually cease to maintain the person's functional ability.

1.  System review: Anti-Parkinson's medications work in a number of ways but generally try to either increase the levels of dopamine (a neurotransmitter) in the brain's striatum or reduce the effect of acetylcholine (an opposing neurotransmitter) in an effort to restore dopamine-acetylcholine balance. We will focus on the dopamine-enhancing drugs.

2.  Drug class information:

    *   General indications: to relieve symptoms and slow disease progress, often drugs are given in combination to enhance effects

    *   General administration routes: medications are given orally

    *   General affects: reduction in symptoms

    *   General adverse effects: nausea and vomiting, abnormal body movements, psychotic symptoms including delusions (fixed irrational or untrue beliefs) and hallucinations (unreal sensory perceptions such as hearing voices or seeing nonexistent things), orthostatic hypotension, arrhythmias (abnormal heart rhythms)

    *   Nursing considerations: instruct to take with food, monitor for side effects, teach safety considerations, r/t blood pressure changes

The following table lists some important and frequently prescribed antiseizure medications:

## Figure 3: Antiseizure medications (for Parkinson's)

| Medication | Specific indications | Specific contraindications | Nursing considerations |
|---|---|---|---|
| Levodopa/carbidopa (Sinemet®) Levodopa was one of the first–stimulates dopamine production | General indications apply | Malignant melanoma history | General nursing considerations apply |
| Pramipexole (Mirapex®) Dopamine receptor agonist | General indications apply | Nothing specific | General nursing considerations apply |
| Ropinirole (Requip®) Dopamine receptor agonist | General indications apply | Similar to Mirapex | General nursing considerations apply |
| Selegiline (Eldepryl®) Inhibits COMT, which metabolizes dopamine | General indications apply | Nothing specific | Most common adverse effect is insomnia |

**An eye on epilepsy**

Anybody know anyone with epilepsy? Between 1%–2% of the population has this seizure disorder. Seizures are the result of abnormal electrical activity in the brain and can result in:

- Generalized rhythmic tonic-clonic movements of the body

- Absence seizures (alteration in level of consciousness)

- Atonic seizures or drop attacks in which children experience a sudden loss of muscle tone and fall

- Status epilepticus

Let's look at a table of common antiseizure medications:

## Figure 4: Antiseizure medications (for epilepsy)

| Medication | Specific indications | Specific contraindications | Nursing considerations |
|---|---|---|---|
| Phenytoin (Dilantin®) One of the oldest and most well-known | Used in all types of seizures | Use with caution in persons with liver disease | Must monitor blood levels to ensure they are sufficient to cause effect but not toxicity; interacts with many medications |
| Carbamazepine (Tegretol®) | All seizures except absence type; bipolar disorder | Persons with blood dyscrasias (abnormal production) | Must monitor blood levels to ensure they are sufficient to cause effect but not toxicity; can cause bone marrow depression with resulting low levels of red blood cells, white blood cells and platelets |
| Valproic Acid (Depakote®) | All seizures; bipolar disorder; migraine headaches | Persons with liver disease | Must monitor blood levels to ensure they are sufficient to cause effect but not toxicity; causes birth defects when taken by pregnant women |
| Gabapentin (Neurontin®) | All seizures; neuropathic pain | Nothing specific | Monitor for dizziness, somnolence, fatigue |
| Topiramate (Topamax®) | All seizures; cluster headaches; neuropathic pain; bulimia (eating disorder) | Caution if renal function impaired | Monitor for somnolence, ataxia (difficulty walking), dizziness, nervousness, double vision, nausea/vomiting |
| Lamotigine (Lamictal®) | All seizures | History of rashes associated with prior use | Can cause life-threatening rashes, dizziness, double vision, nausea/vomiting |

## Peeking in on the peripheral nervous system

We've familiarized ourselves with the central nervous system, so let's turn our attention to the periphery—all those neurons that travel to and from our spinal cord. These nerves are either sympathetic (adrenergic is another term) or parasympathetic (cholinergic). Remember the fight or flight stress response you heard about in biology? Do you recall the counterbalancing response, breed and feed? Prepare for a review. Sympathetic refers to body responses that we would need to fight or run away. Parasympathetic indicates a set of responses that would be useful for breeding and feeding. Learn the specific responses listed below with the help of three peripheral nervous system tips.

**Tip:** If you learn sympathetic first, parasympathetic is just the opposite!

- Sympathetic: vasoconstriction (narrowing of blood vessels to raise blood pressure), increased heart rate, increased respiratory rate, relax gastrointestional (GI) and urinary muscles, dilated pupils, increased sweat, dilated bronchioles in lungs, increased blood flow to skeletal muscles

- Parasympathetic: vasodilation to lower blood pressure, slowed heart rate, slowed respiratory rate, contracted smooth muscle in GI and urinary systems, constricted pupils, decreased sweat, constricted bronchioles, decreased blood flow to skeletal muscles

**Tip:** Agonists stimulate receptors and antagonists inhibit receptors. Normally, both the sympathetic and parasympathetic systems are active and in balance. Sympathetic agonists and parasympathetic antagonists increase the sympathetic response. Parasympathetic agonists and sympathetic antagonists increase the parasympathetic response.

**Tip:** There are four types of sympathetic receptors (alpha 1, alpha 2, beta 1, beta 2) and three types of parasympathetic receptors (muscarinic, nicotinic n, and nicotinic m.) We will focus on muscarinic receptors because they most often are the target for parasympathetic-related medications as well as being responsible for the parasympathetic signs and symptoms experienced by our patients.

The following table gives a quick summary of each receptor and its actions. Medications affecting the peripheral nervous system are all designed to inhibit or enhance the effects of solitary receptors or combinations.

## Figure 5: Receptors and actions

| Receptor type | Location and function |
|---|---|
| Alpha 1 (sympathetic) | Dilates eyes, constricts veins and arterioles (skin, mucous membranes, internal organs), responsible for ejaculation in males, contracts urinary sphincter muscles |
| Alpha 2 (sympathetic) | Inhibits neurotransmitter release in the central nervous system—not an important site for us due to the limited number of medications |
| Beta 1 (sympathetic) | Increases heart rate, increases strength of heart contraction, increases velocity of conduction in the heart's AV node, stimulates renin release in kidney |
| Beta 2 (sympathetic) | Dilates arterioles (heart, lungs, skeletal muscle), dilates bronchi, relaxes uterus, glycogenolysis (released of stored glucose) in liver, enhance contraction in skeletal muscle |
| Muscarinic | Constricts eyes, slows heart and respiration, constricts bronchioles, stimulates GI secretion and motility, stimulates urination, responsible for erection, dilates blood vessels |

Now all you need to do is learn the list of drugs. If you remember the three tips from the previous page, learning which drug does what is easy:

## Common muscarinic agonists

- Bethanechol (prototype)—usually prescribed for urinary retention

- Pilocarpine—used as eye drops, constricts the eye to help drainage of fluids and reduce intraocular pressure

- Acetylcholine—eye drops to constrict the pupil during eye surgery

## Common muscarinic antagonists

- Atropine (prototype)—to treat slow heart rates, dilate pupils, and as an antidote to muscarinic poisoning

- Oxybutynin (Ditropan®)—to treat overactive bladder

- Scopolamine—used in anesthesia and to treat motion sickness

- Dicyclomine (Bentyl®)—treat GI spasm and cramping

## Common adrenergic agonists

- Alpha 1 and 2, Beta 1 and 2—Epinephrine, Ephedrine

- Alpha 1 and Beta 1—Dopamine

## Common adrenergic antagonists

- Alpha 1 and 2—Phentolamine (used to dilate blood vessels as an antidote if adrenergic agonists leak during intravenous infusion)

- Alpha 1—doxazosin, prazosin, terazosin (used to lower blood pressure in both genders, reduce urinary obstruction from prostate enlargement in men)

- Beta 1 and 2—labetalol, nadolol, propranolol, sotalol (reduce blood pressure and slow heart rate)

- Beta 1—metoprolol, esmolol, atenolol (to produce desired heart effects without constricting bronchioles)

As you can see, a careful selection of medications creates the desired response. For example, a beta antagonist (blocker) like propranolol may be a good option for hypertension (elevated blood pressure) because it inhibits sympathetic responses and lowers blood pressure. And an understanding of receptors gives us a clue as to possible side effects. Propranolol also inhibits beta 2 receptors that can cause narrowing of bronchi and bronchioles, which explains why some people on beta blockers for hypertension experience asthma- or wheezing-type symptoms.

Whew! Almost there, don't despair!

We've reviewed the neurological system and examined medications that affect the central component as well as the two branches of the peripheral nervous system. We've looked at the receptors associated with each branch of the peripheral nervous system and decided the important ones for us to remember are alpha 1, beta 1, beta 2 in the sympathetic branch, and muscarinic in the parasympathetic branch. To wrap up, let's take a look at mental health medications.

## A little mental health

First, let's look at a few numbers to give us perspective. Consider these facts:

**Did you know:**

- One percent of the world population has or will have a psychotic disorder called schizophrenia

- Up to 30% of Americans will experience major depression symptoms, and 15% of those really have bipolar (manic-depression) disorder

- Research indicates that anywhere from 2% to 43% (study results widely vary) of children experience diagnosable anxiety disorders at some point before reaching maturity (Townsend)

Clearly, mental health treatment options are needed. Until the late 1950s, there were very few psychotropic medications (drugs that treat mental health conditions). The best way to look at them is in groups, so let's use the following tables. They list examples of the more commonly prescribed drugs in each class.

## Figure 6: Antidepressants

| Medication | Indications | Potential adverse effects |
|---|---|---|
| **Tricyclics**<br>Amitriptyline (Elavil®)<br><br>Imipramine (Tofranil®) | This was the first class of antidepressants; used to treat depression and bipolar disorder | Orthostatic hypotension, sedation, cardiotoxicity, seizures; overdose can be fatal |
| **Selective serotonin reuptake inhibitors**<br><br>Citalopram (Celexa®)<br><br>Escitalopram (Lexapro®)<br><br>Paroxetine (Paxil®)<br><br>Sertraline (Zoloft®) | Newer drugs used for depression, bipolar disorder, eating disorders, anxiety disorders | Weight gain, serotonin syndrome (agitation, confusion, tremors, hyperreflexia, death), withdrawal syndrome, sexual dysfunction |
| **Monoamine oxidase inhibitors (MAOIs)**<br><br>Isocarboxazid (Marplan®)<br><br>Phenelzine (Nardil®)<br><br>Tranylcypromine (Parnate®) | Seldom used because of extensive side effect and drug interaction concerns; used to treat depression | Hypertensive (elevated blood pressure) crisis when eating tyramine-containing foods (yeast extracts, cheese, sausages, and others) |
| **Others**<br><br>Bupropion (Wellbutrin®, Zyban®) | Depression, smoking cessation | Seizures, agitation, headache, dizziness, tachycardia, weight loss |
| Mirtazapine (Remeron®) | Depression | Somnolence, weight gain, cholesterol elevation, dizziness |
| Trazodone (Desyrel®) | Depression, insomnia | Somnolence, hypotension, priapism (prolonged painful erection) |

## Figure 7: Antipsychotics

| Medication | Indications | Potential adverse effects |
|---|---|---|
| **Typical**<br><br>Haloperidol (Haldol®)<br><br>Chlorpromazine (Thorazine®)<br><br>Loxapine (Loxitane®) | Older drugs that are still available but less commonly used; used to treat schizophrenia and psychotic symptoms (hallucinations, delusions) or aggressive behaviors in other disorders | Extrapyramidal effects (dystonia or alterations in muscle tone and spasms, parkinsonism or symptoms just like Parkinson's disease, akathisia or profound restlessness and agitation, and tardive dyskinesia); also can experience neuroleptic malignant syndrome: muscle rigidity, fever, autonomic instability<br><br>Others: anticholinergic effects, orthostatic hypotension, sedation, seizures, sexual dysfunction |
| **Atyptical**<br><br>Olanzapine (Zyprexa®)<br><br>Aripiprazole (Abilify®)<br><br>Quetiapine (Seroquel®)<br><br>Risperidone (Risperdal®) | Newer medications, used for schizophrenia and bipolar disorder | Fewer extrapyramidal effects, although still possible, weight gain, diabetes, agranulocytosis |

**Figure 8: Mood stabilizers**

| Medication | Indications | Potential adverse effects |
|---|---|---|
| Lithium carbonate (Eskalith®)<br><br>Other drugs include antipsychotics and anticonvulsants | Management of bipolar disorder; treatment of mania in bipolar disorders | Nausea, vomiting, diarrhea, thirst, sedation, confusion, convulsions, and death when toxic; must monitor blood levels |

**Figure 9: Anxiolytics/hypnotics**

| Medication | Indications | Potential adverse effects |
|---|---|---|
| **Benzodiazepines**<br>Alprazolam (Xanax®)<br><br>Clonazepam (Klonopin®)<br><br>Diazepam (Valium®)<br><br>Oxazepam (Serax®) | Anxiety, obsessive compulsive disorder, alcohol withdrawal | Abuse potential, somnolence, daytime sedation |

Well, we made it through the neuro and mental health section. Make flash-cards for these drugs to help you learn drug classes, uses, and effects. Also, keep reviewing the receptors until they are second nature. Take a break—briefly—and then let's go on to the cardiovascular system.

## References

"About Parkinson Disease." National Parkinson Web site. Available at *www.parkinson.org/netcommunity/page.aspx?pid=225&srcid=201*. Accessed December 3, 2007.

Katzung, B. (1998). *Basic and Clinical Pharmacology,* 7th ed. Stamford, CT: Appleton and Lange.

Lehne, R. (2007). *Pharmacology for Nursing Care,* 6th ed. St. Louis: Elsevier.

Porth, C. (2004). *Essentials of Pathophysiology,* 6th ed. Philadelphia: Lippincott Williams & Wilkins.

Springhouse (2003). *Professional Guide to Pathophysiology*. Philadelphia: Lippincott Williams & Wilkins.

Townsend, M. (2006). *Psychiatric Mental Health Nursing: Concepts of Care in Evidence-Based Practice,* 5th ed. Philadelphia: F.A. Davis Company.

Wilson, B., Shannon, M., Shields, K. and Stang, C. (2007). *Nurse's Drug Guide 2007*. Upper Saddle River, New Jersey: Prentice Hall.

# Chapter 14

# Put your heart into it: Cardiovascular medications

The task for this lesson is to gain a solid understanding of cardiovascular medications. We will start with a review of basic cardiovascular physiology. Then we will look at specific medications used to treat arrhythmias (abnormal heart rhythms), hypertension (elevated blood pressure), angina (chest pain related to cardiac ischemia), and heart failure. We will also examine drugs used to modify coagulation and lower serum lipid (fat) levels. Are you ready to get to the heart of the matter? (Okay, sorry for the horrendous pun.)

The purpose of the cardiovascular system is to deliver nutrients and oxygen to tissues throughout the body and to transport waste to the organs for metabolism and excretion. The four-chambered heart synchronously contracts to pump blood in two distinct circulation pathways: pulmonic and systemic.

- The pulmonary circulation flows through the right half of the heart, pulmonary artery, pulmonary vein, and the pulmonary capillaries in the lungs. Its purpose is to carry blood to the lungs for gas exchange. It is important to note that we can manipulate its function by making the heart pump faster and slower or stronger and weaker. We can also give medications to dilate (vasodilation) or constrict (vasoconstriction) blood vessels or medications that prevent the formation of clots that hamper gas exchange. The pulmonary circulation is a low pressure system.

- The systemic circulation flows through the left half of the heart, the aorta, the vena cava, and the capillary beds in all the tissues outside of the pulmonary circulation. We can also manipulate systemic circulation by changing the speed and strength of cardiac contraction or by altering the diameter of systemic blood vessels. In addition, drugs may be used to help the body excrete surplus water. Finally, medications are employed to prevent impaired circulation due to fatty buildup and blood clots.

 **Don't forget:** The majority of cardiac symptoms or disease are treated by any combination of the following: altering heart rate, changing the strength of heart contraction, dilating or constricting blood vessels, inhibiting clotting mechanisms, lowering lipid levels, or promoting excretion of water.

## About arrhythmias

The normal heart initiates an electrical impulse in the sinoatrial node that is transmitted to the atrioventricular node and on to the ventricles through the Purkinje fibers. The net effect is atria (upper chambers) that contract just before and help to completely fill the ventricles (lower chambers). Arrhythmias (altered or absent rhythms) tend to be divided into two broad categories: supraventricular (above the ventricles) and ventricular dysrhythmias (abnormal or disturbed rhythm in the ventricles) (Venes, et al.). The heart can be too fast in tachycardia or too slow in bradycardia. Atrial fibrillation, atrial flutter, and paroxysmal atrial tachycardia (sudden and dangerous accelerations of heart rate) are supraventricular disturbances.

Drugs used to treat rhythm disturbances are categorized as sodium channel blockers (class I), beta blockers (class II), potassium channel blockers (class III), calcium channel blockers (class IV), and "other." Class I drugs are further divided into subclasses, but that is more detail than we need to consider here.

The following table lists common antiarrhythmics and their uses and side effects. There are many others, and new ones every year, so the prudent and safe nurse knows and uses reliable information sources. You will be conferring with other healthcare providers, such as physicians and pharmacists, of course, but there are good information sites on the Internet.

 **Click:** Go to *www.drugs.com* as a source of lay and professional information.

**Figure 10: Common antiarrhythmics**

| Medication | Indications | Potential adverse effects |
|---|---|---|
| Quinidine (sodium channel blocker) (Quinaglute®) | Supraventricular and ventricular arrhythmia | Diarrhea, GI upset, tinnitus (ringing ears), dizziness, heart blocks, hypotension |
| Procainamide (sodium channel blocker) (Procan®) | Supraventricular and ventricular arrhythmias | Systemic lupus erythematosis-like syndrome, nausea, hypotension |
| Lidocaine (sodium channel blocker) (Xylocaine®) | Ventricular arrhythmias | Drowsiness, confusion, convulsions, respiratory arrest |
| Propranolol (beta blocker) (Inderal®) | Dysrhythmias due to excess sympathetic stimulus | Bradycardia, hypotension, heart blocks, heart failure, asthma-like symptoms |
| Amiodarone (potassium channel blocker) (Cordarone®) | Life-threatening ventricular dysrhythmias | Pulmonary toxicity, cardiac toxicity, liver toxicity, thyroid toxicity, blurred vision, anorexia, nausea, vomiting; many drug interactions |
| Verapamil (calcium channel blocker) (Calan®) | Reduce ventricular rate in supraventricular arrhythmias | Bradycardia, AV block, hypotension, peripheral edema (limb swelling), constipation |
| Adenosine (other) (Adenocard®) | Stop paroxysmal supraventricular tachycardia | Bradycardia, hypotension, chest discomfort |
| Digoxin (other) (Lanoxin®) | Reduce ventricular rate in supraventricular arrhythmias | Nausea, vomiting, bradycardia, heart block |

## The hype about antihypertensives

Even if your patient's heart is beating strongly in the appropriate rhythm, he or she can be at risk. The patient may develop organ disease (kidney failure, heart enlargement, strokes from altered circulation in the brain) from an elevated blood pressure (hypertension). Our bodies regulate blood pressure through constricting and dilating blood vessels, maintaining appropriate fluid balance, and adjusting the rate and strength of heart contraction. The following table gives examples of medications used to treat hypertension.

## Figure 11: Common antihypertensives

| Medication | Indications | Potential adverse effects |
|---|---|---|
| Verapamil (calcium channel blocker) (Calan®) | Dilates arterioles and has direct effect on heart | Headache, dizziness, constipation, hypotension, bradycardia, tachycardia |
| Prazosin (alpha 1 blocker) (Minipress®) | Prevents vasoconstriction due to alpha 1 stimulation | Dizziness, headache, drowsiness, hypotension, palpitations |
| Lisinopril (angiotensin converting enzyme inhibitor) (Prinivil®) | Prevents vasoconstriction and water retention by inhibiting the formation of angiotensin; may also work to decrease adrenergic outflow from CNS | Hypotension, cough, chest pain, hyperkalemia (elevated serum potassium) |
| Losartan (angiotensin II receptor blocker) (Cozaar®) | Inhibits effects of angiotensin by direct receptor blockade | Dizziness, insomnia, headache, hypotension, muscle cramps, sinusitis |
| Furosemide (loop diuretic) (Lasix®) | Reduce circulating blood volume by producing profound diuresis (water loss by kidneys) | Hypotension, hypokalemia (low serum potassium), dehydration, hearing loss |
| Hydrochlorthiazide (Thiazide diuretic) (Oretic®) | Diuresis (water loss by kidneys) initially; peripheral vasodilating effect over time | As in loop diuretics but less effect, no effect on hearing |
| Propranolol (beta blocker beta 1 and 2) (Inderal®) | Inhibits beta receptors to slow heart rate and reduce vasoconstriction | Hypotension, heart block, heart failure, asthma symptoms |
| Metoprolol (selective beta blocker just beta 1) (Lopressor®) | Inhibits beta receptors to slow heart rate and reduce vasoconstriction | Similar to propranolol but selectively less effect on beta 2 |
| Clonidine (centrally acting alpha 2 agonist) (Catatres®) | Decrease sympathetic outflow from presynaptic nerurons in the brainstem | Sedation, dry mouth, hemolytic anemia, hypotension, constipation |

Again, there are many, many more antihypertensive medications. Consult with other healthcare providers (nurse practitioners, physician assistants, pharmacists) and draw on text or web resources. Check this one out:

 **Click:** For more information on cardiovascular pharmacology concepts, go here: *www.cvpharmacology.com/antihypertensive/antihypertensive.htm.*

## A look at angina

Our next topic in this lesson is the pharmacological treatment of angina, or chest pain due to cardiac ischemia (decreased blood flow to the heart). There are three types of angina: stable (comes on with exertion and is the most common form), unstable (dangerous and unpredictable, can be unrelated to exercise), and variant (Prinzmetal's; occurs in the morning or evening at rest) (National Heart Lung and Blood Institute). We will focus on stable angina.

Now here comes the good part: We have already discussed most of the medications! You have already learned about beta blockers. They help angina by decreasing heart rate and the strength of contraction (contractility). Calcium channel blockers are used to dilate arterioles and decrease heart rate.

The only new class is the nitrates, which essentially are varied formulations of nitroglycerin. Some—such as Nitrostat®, a sublingual (under the tongue) medication—begin to work in seconds and have a very brief half-life, while others are topical patches that help maintain steady blood levels. Here's a look in chart form:

### Figure 12: Angina medications

| Medication | Indications | Potential adverse effects |
|---|---|---|
| Nitrates | Dilates veins, which decreases oxygen need of heart by reducing workload | Hypotension, headache, reflex tachycardia; there must be a nitrate-free period (6-8 hours) during the day in order to prevent tolerance and loss of effect from developing |

## Ace the test on heart failure

Put simply, heart failure is a condition in which the heart is unable to pump sufficiently to meet the body's needs and is characterized by a steadily worsening condition. It can be caused by long-standing hypertension, heart attacks, heavy alcohol use, heart valve disease, and a variety of other conditions. As the pump fails, fluid accumulates in the lungs and body tissues. This impairs breathing and activity tolerance. We have already learned about the drugs used to treat heart failure, but the table below is a good review:

### Figure 13: Heart failure medications

| Medication | Indications | Potential adverse effects |
| --- | --- | --- |
| Diuretics <br>• Loop (furosemide, etc.) <br>• Thiazide (hydrochlorothiazide, etc.) <br>• Potassium sparing (spironolactone, etc.) | Diuresis: Promote excretion of excess body fluid; loop diuretics are the most potent; potassium sparing medications diminish potassium loss | Hypotension, dehydration, potassium wasting with loop and thiazide diuretics—often need to take a potassium supplement; hyperkalemia (too high serum potassium) with potassium sparing medications |
| Angiotensin converting enzyme (ACE) inhibitors: lisinopril, captopril, etc. | Inhibit the conversion of angiotensin I to angiotensin II, causing less vasoconstriction, and suppression of aldosterone, causing less water and sodium retention | Hypotension, cough, chest pain, hyperkalemia |
| Angiotensin receptor II blockers: candesartan, losartan, etc. | Directly block the effect of angiotensin II, similar to ACE inhibitor effect | Dizziness, insomnia, headache, hypotension, muscle cramps, sinusitis; often better tolerated than ACE inhibitors |
| Cardiac glycoside: digoxin | Increase contractility, slow heart rate | Nausea, vomiting, bradycardia, heart block |

# A glance at anticoagulants

How many times have you cut or nicked yourself? Clotting, we'd all have to agree, is essentially a good thing. There are times, however, when our clotting cascade pathway overresponds to a real or perceived threat and runs amok. Most strokes or cerebral vascular accidents are due to clots lodging in arteries and arterioles in the brain (ischemic strokes), and heart attacks are often the result of clots blocking the coronary arteries. Blood clots can develop in the legs as deep vein thromboses and shed small particles that float as emboli to the lungs (pulmonary emboli) where they may cause death.  The table below lists drugs used to prevent excessive coagulation:

## Figure 14: Anticoagulants

| Medication | Indications | Potential adverse effects |
|---|---|---|
| Heparin (unfractionated) | Decreases fibrin formation by inactivating clotting factors; effect must be monitored by lab test; activated partial thromboplastin time, can only be given intravenously or subcutaneously | Hemorrhage, bruising, heparin-induced thrombocytopenia (resulting in extremely low platelets) |
| Low molecular weight heparins (fractionated) | Decreases fibrin formation by inactivating generally only one clotting factor; given subcutaneously | Less risk of hemorrhage but bruising and bleeding still possible |
| Warfarin (Coumadin®) | Decreases fibrin formation by inhibiting formation of vitamin K-dependent clotting factors; can only be given orally; effect must be monitored with prothrombin time (PT) or international normalized ratio (INR) | Slower onset than heparin; counteracted by foods containing vitamin K |
| Aspirin (inhibits platelet aggregation) | Inhibits cyclooxygenase | GI bleeding or hemorrhagic stroke |
| Clodpidogrel (Plavix®) (adenosine diphosphate receptor antagonist) | An antiplatelet aggregation agent approved for use to prevent ischemic strokes | Abdominal pain, GI bleeding, hemorrhagic stroke |

## Lastly, lipid levels

Hang on, just one more topic for today. How can we prevent that dietary fat from giving our patient that big MI (myocardial infarction or heart attack)? First things first: We need to tell our patient to put down that double cheese-burger smothered with mayo and topped with bacon. There are no medications that will prevent suicide by food. Having said that, it is clear that appropriate medications, coupled with a faithful effort to modify lifestyle, will greatly diminish our patient's cardiovascular risk.

We are concerned about total cholesterol, low density lipoprotein cholesterol (LDL), high density lipoprotein cholesterol (HDL), and triglycerides (TG). We do require some cholesterol to make myelin in the brain and along axons. It is also the basic framework our body uses to build sex hormones and adrenal corticoids. Even if we were able to eat a diet entirely free of cholesterol, our bodies would make it. But too much dietary intake or a metabolic predisposition toward overproduction does contribute to athero-sclerosis and heart attacks. The goal is to lower our total cholesterol, triglyc-erides, and LDL while increasing our proportion of HDL. Our last table in this class gives examples of medications used to lower fats:

## Figure 15: Fat-lowering medications

| Medication | Indications | Potential adverse effects |
|---|---|---|
| HMG-CoA reductase inhibitors, or "Statins": pravastatin, atorvastatin, lovastatin and others | Inhibits an enzyme: HMG-CoA reductase to lower LDL and triglycerides | Nausea, diarrhea, abdominal pain, hepatotoxicity, myopathy (damage to muscle); can't be taken during pregnancy or by people with liver disease |
| Niacin (Niacor®) | Cofactor in a fat reduction reaction that reduces total cholesterol, triglycerides, and LDL; raises HDL | Headache, flushing, hepatotoxicity; effective doses almost always produce side effects; can be purchased OTC; can't be taken by people with liver disease or gout |
| Fibrates: gemfibrozil, fenofibrate | Reduces LDL and triglycerides and raises HDL by blocking lipolysis of triglycerides and hepatic reuptake of fats | Can't be taken by people with gallbladder, liver, or kidney disease; can cause abdominal pain, muscle cramps, rash, hyperglycemia (elevated blood sugar) |
| Bile acid sequestrants: colesevelam, cholestyramine | Prevents bile acids from being reabsorbed in the intestine and leading to formation of more cholesterol | Constipation, inhibit absorption of multiple medications |

Well done, people! We've made it through the cardiovascular lesson.

**Watch out:** Just a note of caution here: One time through is not enough. Now would be a great time to do a quick review of the mental training and learning strategies in Chapters 3 and 4. Take all of this information in small bites and return to it often.

**Tip:** Consider spending the first 10%–20% of each study period doing a quick review of the important points in earlier lessons. Now, let's all take a suggestion from an earlier lesson and meditate for a few minutes, relax, recharge, create a few moments of emptiness, and get ready for respiratory pharmacology.

## References

"Cardiovascular Pharmacology Concepts." Antihypertensive Drugs. Available at *www.cvpharmacology.com/antihypertensive/antihypertensive.htm*. Accessed December 7, 2007.

"Drugs.com." Available at *www.drugs.com*. Accessed December 7, 2007.

Lehne, R. (2007). *Pharmacology for Nursing Care*, 6th ed. St. Louis: Elsevier.

Porth, C. (2004). *Essentials of Pathophysiology*, 6th ed. Philadelphia: Lippincott Williams & Wilkins.

Springhouse (2003). *Professional Guide to Pathophysiology*. Philadelphia: Lippincott Williams & Wilkins.

Venes, D. and Thomas, C. (eds) (2001). *Taber's Cylcopedic Medical Dictionary*. Philadelphia: F.A. Davis Company.

"What is Angina?" National Heart Lung and Blood Institute. Available at *www.nhlbi.nih.gov/health/dci/Diseases/Angina/Angina_WhatIs.html*. Accessed December 7, 2007.

Wilson, B., Shannon, M., Shields, K., and Stang, C. (2007). *Nurse's Drug Guide 2007*. Upper Saddle River, New Jersey: Prentice Hall.

# Chapter 15

# Revelations on respirator system medications

## Fighting colds and allergies

Ah . . . chooo! Excuse me. In Michigan, where I am writing this, physicians and nurse practitioners have a joke: Everyone in the state either has allergies or respiratory infections or is about to get them. There is a ton of truth to that—and not just in Michigan.

 **Did you know:** According to the National Institute of Allergy and Infectious Diseases (NIAID), a part of the National Institute of Health, over the course of the year, people suffer approximately 1 billion colds. A pretty impressive number since the number of people in the United States today is 303,571,147, according to the U.S. Census. That's a rough average of 3.5 colds per person each year.

There are no medications yet that cure colds. These self-limited viral infections get better in seven to 10 days with or without medications.

Respiratory allergies are also fairly common. According to the NIAID, an estimated 35 million Americans suffer from the symptoms of upper respiratory tract allergies. There are many symptoms common to both allergies and colds: rhinorrhea (runny nose), narrowed airways, swollen mucosal membranes, and so on. The following tables give examples of medications used to treat symptoms. Remember, these are not exhaustive lists but rather commonly employed important representatives from each category.

## Aim high with antihistamines

Histamine is a substance our body produces from the amino acid histidine, which acts on histamine 1 (H1) receptors to cause dilation of blood vessels, bronchoconstriction (narrowed airways), increased mucus production, tissue swelling, and itching. Histamine can also stimulate histamine 2 (H2) receptors to increase gastric secretions (Venes, D., et al., and Lehne). As we would expect, antihistamines inhibit those responses. Antihistamines come in two flavors: first generation and second generation. The primary difference is that the original antihistamines, first generation, did relieve symptoms but almost invariably caused significant sedation. Second-generation medications arose from efforts to create drugs with less sedation and other side effects.

The table below gives examples of older first-generation and more recent second-generation medications:

**Figure 16: Antihistamines**

| Medication | Indications | Potential adverse effects |
|---|---|---|
| **1st generation**<br><br>Chlorpheniramine (Chlor-Trimeton® and other brands) Diphenhydramine (Benadryl®) Hydroxyzine (Vistaril®) | Mild to moderate allergy symptoms relief, severe allergies, cold symptoms (rhinorrhea, itching, tissue swelling), motion sickness, insomnia | Sedation leading to impaired memory or accidents; cannot be used along with alcohol or other sedatives; dizziness, fatigue, impaired coordination, nausea, dry mouth, urinary retention |
| **2nd generation**<br><br>Fexofenadine (Allegra®) Loratadine (Claritin®) Certirizine (Zyrtec®) | As above except insomnia | As above except less sedation; headache, potential heart arrhythmias |

## A dip into decongestants

These medications help to relieve the nasal stuffiness associated with colds. They do not ease the runny nose, sneezing, or itching. Let's look at a couple of typical drugs:

### Figure 17: Decongestants

| Medication | Indications | Potential adverse effects |
|---|---|---|
| Oxymetazoline (Afrin®, Neo-Synephrine®)

Pseudoephedrine (Sudafed®) | Stimulate alpha 1 receptors on nasal blood vessels, which causes vasoconstriction | Restlessness, agitation, insomnia, irritability, hypertension, stroke, tachyphylaxis (need more and more drug to achieve the same effect) can develop with prolonged use of oxymetazoline |

## Antitussives as an alternative

"Doctor, I have a cough. Can I have some morphine please?" Don't laugh, the most effective cough suppressants (antitussives) are opioids. A physician, however, is unlikely to be amused, should you ask, or prescribe morphine. Here are some typical meds:

### Figure 18: Antitussives

| Medication | Indications | Potential adverse effects |
|---|---|---|
| Codeine | Opioid that acts in the CNS to elevate the cough threshold; an interesting note: The amount needed to suppress cough is much smaller than that needed to give pain relief, so abuse potential is low | Generally well tolerated, nausea, vomiting, sedation |
| Dextromethorphan (DM-cough) | Opioid-derivative but lacking in narcotic properties in normal doses; acts in the CNS | Dizziness, drowsiness, central nervous system depression |
| Benzonatate (Tessalon®) | Similar chemically to a local anesthetic believed to decrease the sensitivity of respiratory tract stretch receptors | Must be swallowed whole to avoid mouth and pharyngeal anesthesia |

## The effectiveness of expectorants

Expectorants are substances that are intended to help the sufferer clear accumulated secretions. They stimulate tissues to produce increased and looser secretions, but their effectiveness is unproven. Some clinicians have advocated that increased fluid intake is just as effective at helping to loosen and clear secretions.

## A grasp on glucocorticoids

Glucocorticoids, or steroids, are not characteristically used to treat colds. They are more often employed to treat chronic allergy symptoms. This table lists widespread nasal medications. We will consider other routes in our asthma and chronic obstructive pulmonary disease (COPD) discussion.

### Figure 19: Nasal medications

| Medication | Indications | Potential adverse effects |
|---|---|---|
| Beclomethasone (Beconase®)  Budesonide (Rhinocort®)  Triamcinolone (Nasacort®) | Reduces the major inflammation symptoms (congestion, itching, sneezing, rhinorrhea) | Generally well tolerated with few side effects if taken appropriately; nasal drying, sore throat, epistaxis (bloody nose) |

# A deeper battle with breathing

Let's turn our attention to deeper respiratory problems. Asthma and chronic obstructive pulmonary disease are great examples of common conditions where typical respiratory medications are brought into play. Examining these diseases will enhance our understanding of the medications.

Asthma is a condition characterized by bronchoconstriction and inflammation of respiratory membranes. It is not a benign condition. Sufferers experience intermittent attacks or acute episodes during which symptoms worsen and can become life threatening.

**Did you know:** The Centers for Disease Control and Prevention (CDC) estimates 15.7 million adults and 6.5 million children currently have asthma. The CDC also reports 1.3 people out of every 100,000 die each year from asthma.

Chronic obstructive pulmonary disease is the fourth leading cause of death in the United States. The CDC states that 41.5 out of every 100,000 people will die from COPD each year. COPD is a group of respiratory conditions characterized by chronic obstruction of airflow in the pulmonary airways that can lead to enlargement of airspaces and destruction of lung tissue (Porth).

Treatment for both of these disorders is aimed at reducing airway obstruction, decreasing secretions, and limiting the body's inflammatory response. Frequently used medications are listed in the following tables:

### Figure 20: Bronchodilators (all of which are used in both asthma and COPD)

| Medication | Indications | Potential adverse effects |
|---|---|---|
| Albuterol (Proventil®, Ventolin®) | Short-acting beta 2 agonist bronchodilator used for immediate relief: the "rescue" medication; given as a aerosolized mist or in with a pocket-sized inhaler | Palpitations, tremor, nervousness, hypertension or hypotension, tachycardia |
| Levalbuterol (Xopenex®) | Short-acting beta 2 agonist that is the active component of albuterol; given as mist | Similar to albuterol but less adverse effects at equivalent doses |
| Salmeterol (Serevent®) | Long-acting beta 2 agonist; used as a preventative; not effective as a rescue med for acute breathing difficulty | Dizziness, headache, tremor, respiratory arrest (rare) |
| Ipratropium (Atrovent®) | Anticholinergic, blocks muscarinic receptors and causes bronchodilation; less effective than beta 2 agonists, but useful in combination with them; administered as a mist or as a spray inhaler | Dry mouth, pharyngeal irritation |
| Theophylline (Theo-Dur®) | Methylxanthine that causes bronchodilation by relaxing smooth muscle; typically administered in long-acting oral forms | Must monitor blood levels; nausea, vomiting, cardiac dysrhythmias, convulsions, death |

## Figure 21: Anti-inflammatory medications

| Medication | Indications | Potential adverse effects |
|---|---|---|
| Glucocorticoids: prednisone, methylprednisolone, dexamethasone | Mimic the natural glucocorticoids produced by the adrenal gland to reduce inflammation; can be administered orally or intravenously for systemic effect; glucocorticoids can also be inhaled for more a localized response and fewer systemic side effects; used in both asthma and COPD | Few with short-term use other than hyperglycemia, euphoria, psychosis; long-term use: heart failure, muscle weakness, osteoporosis, cushingoid features, diminished immune response, delayed wound healing, cataracts, and others |
| Leukotriene modifiers: montelukast, zafirlukast | Reduce effect of leukotrienes, which are compounds that promote bronchospasm and mucous production | Headache, GI disturbances, hepatic toxicity, elevated levels of other medications due to metabolism site competition |
| Cromolyn | Safest asthma drug; used to prevent attacks by suppressing the inflammatory response; administered through inhalation | Occasional cough or bronchospasm |
| Omalizumab (Xolair®) | New monoclonal antibody that binds to IgE receptors and inhibits immune response; given as a subcutaneous injection | Anaphylaxis (profound allergic reaction), joint pain, upper respiratory infections, rash, earache |

## Bringing it home

Let's recap a bit. We've looked at the medications used to treat upper respiratory disorders such as allergy symptoms and colds. We saw that usual pharmacologic approaches for colds were aimed toward reducing cold symptoms such as cough and congestion as patients waited for the infection to run its course. The upper respiratory allergy treatments aimed to reduce the inflammatory responses.

Then, we looked at two common respiratory diseases—asthma and COPD—as a framework to examine the effects of other medications.

One last point: There are new drugs approved each year because these are common conditions that afflict huge numbers of people. Books are sometimes outdated even as they are published, so remain current through electronic resources.

 **Click:** Visit the U.S. Food and Drug Administration site (*www.fda.gov*) and enter one of the drugs we've considered here in the search feature. You'll find enormous amounts of great information.

# References

"Airborne Allergens: Something in the Air." U.S. Department of Health and Human Services. Available at *http://www3.niaid.nih.gov/healthscience/healthtopics/allergicDiseases/PDF/airborne_allergens.pdf*. Accessed December 9, 2007.

"Asthma Fast Stats." Centers for Disease Control and Prevention. Available at *www.cdc.gov/nchs/fastats/asthma.htm*. Accessed December 9, 2007.

"Common Cold." National Institute of Allergy and Infectious Diseases. Available at *http://www3.niaid.nih.gov/healthscience/healthtopics/colds/overview.htm*. Accessed December 9, 2007.

"Chronic Obstructive Pulmonary Disease." Centers for Disease Control and Prevention. Available at *www.cdc.gov/nceh/airpollution/copd/copdfaq.htm*. Accessed January 7, 2008.

Lehne, R. (2007). *Pharmacology for Nursing Care*, 6th ed. St. Louis: Elsevier.

Porth, C. (2004). *Essentials of Pathophysiology*, 6th ed. Philadelphia: Lippincott Williams & Wilkins.

Springhouse. (2003). *Professional Guide to Pathophysiology*. Philadelphia: Lippincott Williams & Wilkins.

U.S. Census Bureau. Available at *www.census.gov*. Accessed December 11, 2007.

Venes, D. and Thomas, C. (eds) (2001). *Taber's Cylcopedic Medical Dictionary*. Philadelphia: F.A. Davis Company.

Wilson, B., Shannon, M., Shields, K., and Stang, C. (2007). *Nurse's Drug Guide 2007*. Upper Saddle River, New Jersey: Prentice Hall.

# Chapter 16

# The goods on gastrointestinal and renal medications

This lesson will feature a quick but important tour of drugs used to treat gastrointestinal (GI) and urological disorders. Each of these topics could be an entire lesson, but the important consideration for us is to build a basic familiarity that enables us to learn general indications, mechanisms, and undesired possible outcomes.

 **Don't forget:** This is a great time to restate an important nursing standard: Anytime you administer a drug you never or seldom give, you MUST (sorry for shouting) look it up in a detailed drug guide that lists all of the indications, dosage ranges, contraindications, and possible adverse effects.

Let's move on to our first topic.

## Chow time: Appetite stimulants and suppressants

Most of us probably don't need to worry about stimulating our appetites. According to the Centers for Disease Control and Prevention, more than 66% of Americans are overweight, and 32% are grossly overweight or obese. Some people do benefit from appetite suppressants, but appetite stimulants are useful for those with chronic conditions that cause anorexia (diminished appetite) or cachexia (severe malnutrition and wasting). The following table lists common examples of each:

## Figure 22: Appetite stimulants and suppressants

| Medication | Indications | Potential adverse effects |
|---|---|---|
| Megestrol (Megace®) | Progestin related hormone given to stimulate appetite; given orally | Vaginal bleeding, breast tenderness, weight gain; give with food if gastric distress occurs |
| Dronabinol (Marinol®) | Derivative from THC, the active ingredient in marijuana; stimulates appetite but mechanism is unclear; given orally to stimulate appetite and decrease chemotherapy associated nausea | Drowsiness, psychologic high, dizziness, anxiety, impaired coordination |
| Diethylpriopion (Tenuate®) | A sympathomimetic amine with fewer amphetamine-type side effects, thought to directly act on the CNS to reduce appetite | Rash, muscle pain, mild euphoria, nervousness, palpitations, tachycardia, impotence |
| Sibutramine (Meridia®) | Selective serotonin reuptake inhibitor; also inhibits norepinephrine and dopamine reuptake | Joint aches, headache, dry mouth, depression, nervousness, dizziness, abdominal pain, increased appetite |

## Fight the pain with peptic ulcer medications

Peptic ulcers are lesions in the mucosal membrane that develop in the lower esophagus, stomach, pylorus, duodenum, or jejunum (Springhouse). They are most often caused by an *H. pylori* bacterial infection, use of nonsteroidal anti-inflammatory drugs, or hypersecretory conditions. The drugs listed in the following table were chosen to represent the various classes of medications that need to be considered when designing a treatment plan for someone with a peptic ulcer. The physician may need to prescribe one or more of the following:

- Antibiotics to help kill the bacteria

- Medications to reduce gastric secretions

- Medications to protect the injured mucosal membrane

- Medications to neutralize secretions

**Figure 23: Peptic ulcer medications**

| Medication | Indications | Potential adverse effects |
|---|---|---|
| Penicillin antibiotic: Amoxicillin (Amoxicillin®) | Attacks *H. pylori* and kills it by rupturing the cell wall | Is a penicillin and cannot be taken by those with penicillin allergy, diarrhea |
| Histamine 2 antagonist: Famotidine (Pepcid®) | Blocks histamine 2 receptors, thus reducing the volume and acidity of gastric secretions | Headache, diarrhea, constipation, drowsiness, dizziness; paranoid psychosis with accumulation or in elderly |
| Proton pump inhibitor: Omeprazole (Prilosec®) | Inhibits the parietal cell pump that pumps gastric acid into the GI tract | Headache, fatigue, dizziness, decreased liver function, rash |
| Barrier Sucralfate (Carafate®) | Reacts with stomach secretions to form a paste that adheres to ulcerated areas | Constipation, gastric discomfort, nausea |
| Antacid Aluminum Hydroxide, Magnesium Hydroxide, Calcium Carbonate (Amphojel®, Milk of Magnesia®, Tums®) | Chemicals that react with and neutralize gastric acid | Diarrhea, constipation, nausea, electrolyte imbalance, toxicity from magnesium or aluminum depending on agent chosen |

# Let's learn about laxatives and antidiarrheals

First, we need to be clear about our definitions. We are going to define constipation as decreased stool frequency and a condition where the fecal mass is hard or difficult to expel. Diarrhea will be defined as passing fluid or unformed stools (Venes, D., et al.). Before any medications are employed, we must try to ascertain the cause of either condition. For example, constipation may be the result of insufficient fluid intake or a side effect associated with opioid pain medication. Diarrhea may be the result of a bacterial infection or a diet change. The appropriate intervention needs to take place, as giving an antidiarrheal to a person with a bacterial infection may significantly worsen the patient's condition. The following table lists common medications given to relieve these symptoms:

## Figure 24: Laxatives and antidiarrheals

| Medication | Indications | Potential adverse effects |
|---|---|---|
| Loperamide (Imodium®) | Inhibits peristalsis by direct action on intestinal muscles; an opioid related to meperidine, it is given to treat diarrhea | Drowsiness, fatigue, constipation, CNS depression, toxic megacolon (dilated colon due to accumulated stool; may perforate bowel wall) |
| Diphenoxylate (Lomotil®) | Synthetic opioid; only available with atropine added to discourage abuse; given to treat diarrhea | Drowsiness, dizziness, nausea, vomiting, urinary retention, toxic megacolon |
| Bisacodyl (Dulcolax®) | Promotes intestinal epithelium permeability to increase lumen fluid volume; given as laxative to promote passage of stool | As with all laxatives, must be certain no bowel obstruction exists, diarrhea, cramping, abdominal pain, electrolyte imbalance |
| Docusate Sodium (Colace®) | Detergent action lowers surface tension and allows water and fats to penetrate stool; given as a stool softener | Mild abdominal cramping, nausea |
| Psyllium (Metamucil®) | A refined fiber that adds bulk to stool; given to treat constipation | Must be given with sufficient water to prevent esophageal or bowel obstruction, nausea, vomiting, cramping, diarrhea; decreases absorption of other medications |

# Stomach churning? Try antiemetics

These medications are given to ease nausea and reduce emesis (vomiting) by various mechanisms. It is important to determine the cause of nausea and vomiting prior to employing medications. Here are some commonly used medications illustrating the range of mechanisms.

## Figure 25: Antiemetics

| Medication | Indications | Potential adverse effects |
|---|---|---|
| Ondansetron (Zofran®)<br><br>Granisetron (Kytril®) | Serotonin antagonists that inhibit the chemoreceptor trigger zone (CTZ) in the brain and vagal components of the vomiting reflex; given to prevent nausea and vomiting associated with chemotherapy or postoperative nausea and vomiting; given oral or IV | Dizziness, headache, sedation, diarrhea, elevation in liver enzymes |
| Dexamethasone (Decadron®) | Glucocorticoid; given oral or IV off label to relieve nausea and vomiting associated with chemotherapy | Vertigo, headaches, fluid/electrolyte disturbances, masking signs of infection, impaired wound healing, bruising, hyperglycemia |
| Prochlorperazine (Compazine®)<br><br>Droperidol (Inapsine®) | Dopamine antagnoist; block emetic effects on CTZ<br><br>Prochlorperazine only—Given orally, IV or IM (intramuscularly)<br><br>Droperidol only—Given IV or IM | Drowsiness, dizziness, extrapyramidal reactions (akathisia, dystonia, parkinsonism) |
| Dimenhydrinate (Dramamine®) | Antihistamine; precise action not known but thought to inhibit cholinergic activity | Drowsiness, headache, insomnia, restlessness, nervousness, dry mouth, constipation, difficulty urinating |
| Scopolamine | Anticholinergic action in CNS to reduce nausea and vomiting associated with motion sickness; administered as patch placed behind the ear | Drowsiness, dry mouth and throat, local irritation, tolerance may develop with continued use |

## Wrapping up with renal medications

We are going to finish up this lesson with renal medications. Remember that the kidney is the primary organ responsible for fluid and electrolyte balance. It also is the chief excretory organ and helps to maintain acid-base balance in the body. Recall that in an earlier lesson we examined sympathetic and parasympathetic receptors that influenced urination and became aware that drugs are used to stimulate or block those receptors. In Chapter 18, we will see how antimicrobial medications treat infections including urinary infections. Just recently, we saw how particular medications help rid the body of excess water during our discussion of heart failure. Let's consider those once more in a bit more detail.

First, we need to call to mind a few details about renal physiology. The nephron is the basic functional unit of the kidney; it is where all the action takes place. Each nephron has a glomerulus and a tubule. The glomerulus is a cluster of capillaries and is surrounded by Bowman's capsule, the bulbous end of the tubular collecting system. It's important to note that water and sodium are absorbed in different ratios and rates at various points along the tubule. Diuretics (medications promoting water loss through the kidney) acting at particular points along the tubule produce varying effects. Also, keep in mind that water follows sodium. This means that drugs that block reabsorption of sodium also prevent reabsorption of water. Patients also need to know that an increased dietary sodium intake increases water retention (because . . . water follows sodium).

The following table lists important medications illustrating these effects:

## Figure 26: Renal medications

| Medication | Indications | Potential adverse effects |
|---|---|---|
| **Thiazide**<br><br>Hydrochlorothiazide | Inhibits reabsorption of sodium (consequently water, too) and chloride in the early portion of the distal convoluted tubule; produces moderate fluid loss | Dehydration, hypotension, hypergly-cemia (elevated blood sugar), hypo-kalemia (low serum potassium levels), hyponatremia (low serum sodium levels), hypochloremia (low serum chloride levels); hypercalcemia |
| **Loop diuretics**<br><br>Furosemide (Lasix®)<br><br>Bumetamide (Bumex®) | Most effective diuretics; they act on the ascending loop of Henle to block sodium (consequently, water) and chloride reabsorption; all of these drugs can be given oral or IV, but the intravenous route produces a more pronounced effect; given for pulmonary edema, heart fail-ure, and other fluid overload situa-tions unresponsive to thiazides | Dehydration, hypotension, hypergly-cemia, hypokalemia, hyponatremia, hypochloremia—all of which are greater with loop than thiazide meds; can also cause hearing loss especially when given with other ototoxic drugs |
| **Potassium-sparing diuretics**<br><br>Spironolactone (Aldactone®)<br><br>Triamterene (Dyrenium®) | Produces mild diuresis, used to diminish potassium loss<br><br>Spironolactone only—Blocks the action of aldosterone (from adrenal gland)<br><br>Triamterene only—Directly inhibits exchange of sodium and potassium | Hyperkalemia (elevated serum potas-sium level); sprionolactone can also cause gynecomastia, drowsiness, headache, confusion, and gastrointes-tinal distress |

## Freshen up before we move forward

You made it though GI and renal, not that there were any doubts! We looked at medications that promote or inhibit appetite, and medications that treat-ed constipation and diarrhea. We examined the treatment for peptic ulcers and medications for nausea and vomiting. Then the lesson finished with a discussion of diuretics.

 **Don't forget:** Why don't we dust off some study tips here before we move on? Remember lecturing the dog (or your kid, or an empty room)? This unit would be great for that! Whenever you have very detailed information or, as in this case, a sizable chunk of seemingly disparate items, giving a lecture will help you identify the information you really know and the remainder that needs a bit more effort.

**Don't forget:** Now is also the time to study with a friend or group. Ask each other questions, such as:

- Tell me the differences between thiazide and loop diuretics.

- What mix of meds might you expect the doctor to order for a peptic ulcer and why?

Remember to do a little pharm every day! That's the way to keep it in your brain!

## References

"Overweight Fast Stats." Centers for Disease Control and Prevention. Available at *www.cdc.gov/nchs/fastats/overwt.htm*. Accessed December 9, 2007.

Lehne, R. (2007). *Pharmacology for Nursing Care*, 6th ed. St. Louis: Elsevier.

Porth, C. (2004). *Essentials of Pathophysiology*, 6th ed. Philadelphia: Lippincott Williams & Wilkins.

Springhouse. (2003). *Professional Guide to Pathophysiology*. Philadelphia: Lippincott Williams & Wilkins.

Venes, D. and Thomas, C. (eds) (2001). *Taber's Cylcopedic Medical Dictionary*. Philadelphia: F.A. Davis Company.

Wilson, B., Shannon, M., Shields, K., and Stang, C. (2007). *Nurse's Drug Guide 2007*. Upper Saddle River, New Jersey: Prentice Hall.

# Chapter 17

# Let's hone in on hormones

The hormones in our endocrine system are miraculous things. Itsy-bitsy, barely measurable amounts of these powerful agents wield the power that regulates our growth, tissue repair, metabolism, stress response, and reproduction, among other things. For example, compare the difference between a prepubescent 10-year-old and a mature (maybe?) 18-year-old adult: The difference is due almost entirely to hormonal influence. This lesson will reflect on selected hormonal pathways and the medications used to treat the disorders that afflict them.

## Rapid review

First, let's do a quick review. Hormones are diverse creatures and can be anything from single amino acids to fantastically complex lipids and proteins (Porth). They work by interacting with receptors, which, in turn, influence cellular processes to create specific enzymes or proteins. These are the substances that produce the desired effects. Typically, there is also a feedback loop, which modulates hormone production.

Perhaps an illustration would be helpful: Imagine a young male consumed with the desire to bulk up and be the best athlete in his particular sport. He decides male hormone supplementation (an illicit but readily available option) is the way to go and takes testosterone in doses several thousand times the amount normally produced by his testes. Over time, his own intrinsic testosterone production will cease, and his testes will atrophy and wither.

Let's look at some common diseases and conditions encountered daily by practicing nurses. We will examine diabetes, abnormal thyroid hormone production, and adrenal gland dysfunction. Then we will have a brief conversation about hormone replacement therapy. Ready? Great, let's get started!

## Dealing with diabetes

**Click:** The National Diabetes Information Clearinghouse (NDIC) found at *www.diabetes.niddk.nih.gov/dm/pubs/statistics* is a stunning information source on the topic.

**Did you know:** Data collectors at the NDIC found that 20.8 million people in this country, about 7% of the population, have diabetes. There are 6.2 million unaware they have the disease.

Let's take a quick, where-the-rubber-hits-the-road look at diabetes. Insulin is a protein our body uses to regulate glucose metabolism and is produced in the Beta cells (not the same as the beta receptors we examined in the peripheral nervous system) of the pancreas. Our bodies cannot transport glucose into cells without insulin, so insufficient hormone production leads to high serum glucose levels and horrendous complications. Imagine a diabetic person whose blood sugars are uncontrolled and persistently elevated. Over time, he or she will most likely develop visual deterioration and blindness due to retinopathy, renal failure because of vascular changes, impaired peripheral circulation leading to nonhealing ulcers of the extremities (a major cause of amputations), and decreased ability to fight infections—all of which practically guarantee disability and premature death.

Diabetes comes in two forms: Type I and Type II. Those with Type I fail to produce insulin and require insulin replacement. Those with Type II produce insufficient amounts of insulin and may have resistance to it. Thus, our medication interventions then are designed to do one or several of the following:

- Replace insulin

- Promote insulin production

- Decrease insulin resistance

- Inhibit release of stored glucose in the body

- Alter absorption of nutrients

Let's look at a few common examples:

## Figure 27: Oral diabetes medications

| Medication | Mechanisms | Potential adverse effects |
|---|---|---|
| **Sulfonylureas:** can be used only in people with some pancreatic production of insulin (Type II diabetic) Glipizide (Glucotrol®) Glyburide (DiaBeta®) Glimepiride (Amaryl®) | Stimulates the pancreas to produce more insulin | Hypoglycemia (blood sugar level too low resulting in cognitive impairments, sweating, anxiety, unconsciousness, death) |
| **Alpha-glucosidase inhibitors:** can be used by both Type I and Type II diabetics Acarbose (Precose®) Miglitol (Glyset®) | Slow carbohydrate digestion | Abdominal cramps, increased stomach "gurgling" (borborygmus), intestinal gas (flatus) |
| **Meglitinides:** can be used only by Type II diabetics Repanglinide (Prandin®) Nateglinide (Starlix®) | Stimulates pancreatic insulin production | Hypoglycemia |
| **Biguanides:** only one drug in this class so far, can be used by Type I and II diabetics Metformin (Glucophage®) | Decreases glucose production by the liver, stimulates muscles to increase use of sugar | Nausea, diarrhea, decreased appetite, rare lactic acidosis |
| **Thiazolidinediones:** can be used by Type I and II diabetics Rosiglitazone (Avandia®) Pioglitazone (Actos®) | Decrease resistance to insulin | Hypoglycemia; increase in lipids; possible increased risk of heart failure |

### Injected medications

The injected medications are primarily insulin and modified insulins. Most need to be injected subcutaneously (into the fatty layer beneath the skin of the abdomen, thighs, and upper arms), but regular insulin can also be administered intravenously. Originally, insulin was obtained by processing beef and pork pancreas glands but currently is produced through recombinant DNA technology. It is important for the nurse to remember that the injected insulin will work whether or not the patient eats; it can cause profound hypoglycemia and death if the serum glucose is too low.

**Figure 28: Injected diabetes medications**

| Medication | Mechanisms | Potential adverse effects |
|---|---|---|
| Regular insulin (short-acting): the prototype; begins to work in 30–60 minutes; has a peak effect between 1–5 hours and lasts a total of 6–10 hours; typically given before a meal or to treat intermittent rises in blood sugar and to supplement longer acting forms | All insulins act by serving as a substitute for insufficient intrinsic insulin production | hypoglycemia |
| Rapid-acting insulins: begin to work in 10–15 minutes and last only 3–5 hours; are particularly useful when administered right before a meal or to treat blood sugar elevations<br>Insulin lispro (Humalog®)<br>Insulin aspart (Novolog®)<br>Insulin glulisine (Apidra®) | | |
| Intermediate insulins: begin to work in 1–2 hours, peak at 6–12 hours and last up to 24 hours; these are used twice daily to provide a base blood insulin level | | |
| Long-acting insulins: older types such as Ultralente begin to work in 4–8 hours, peak in 16–18 hours, and last for up to 36 hours.<br>Insulin glargine (Lantus®): a fantastic new insulin that has taken the place of older long-acting insulins and lasts for 24 hours without peak effects; predictable! | | |
| Insulin detemir (Levemir®): not as long-acting as glargine; may still need to be given twice daily | | |

# Taking apart the thyroid

The thyroid gland straddles the larynx in the neck and produces thyroid hormone in two forms: T3 and T4. Thyroid hormone stimulates metabolism. A patient producing inadequate amounts (hypothyroidism) would have a decreased metabolic rate, elevated cholesterol levels, fatigue, somnolence (sleepiness), weight gain, bradycardia, decreased cardiac output, cold intolerance, and myxedema (facial swelling). Hypothyroidism can develop as a result of autoimmune disease, medications, a congenital defect, or decreased pituitary function.

Persons with increased thyroid function experience increased metabolic rates, exophthalmos (bulging eyes), restlessness, irritability, anxiety, heat intolerance, increased cardiac output, tachycardia, and weight loss. Hyperthyroidism arises from Graves' disease, tumors, or overmedication with thyroid hormone. The table below lists some of the drugs often used to treat these conditions.

## Figure 29: Thyroid medications

| Medication | Mechanisms | Potential adverse effects |
| --- | --- | --- |
| Levothyroxine (synthetic) or thyroid hormone (from animals): thyroid hormone either synthetically produced (preferred) or derived from animal thyroid glands | Mimics natural thyroid function | Essentially none if proper amounts are administered; can show signs of hyperthyroidism or hypothyroidism if dose incorrect |
| Radioactive iodine: used to treat Graves' disease | Destroys thyroid tissue as the gland concentrates the iodine within it | Goal is to decrease thyroid hormone production without completely destroying gland; hyporthyroidism agranulocytosis, hypothyroidism |
| Propylthiouracil: used to treat Graves' disease | Blocks thyroid hormone synthesis; process takes up to 12 weeks before thyroid levels approach normal | |
| Potassium Iodide (Lugol's Solution, SSKI)—used to treat Graves' disease by reducing thyroid production in preparation for thyroid surgery | High iodine concentration suppresses thyroid production | Headache, nasal inflammation, burning in mouth, altered taste |

## Picking apart the pituitary and adrenal

You can live without your pancreas if you are committed to taking insulin and the digestive enzymes the pancreas produces. If your thyroid doesn't function, no worries—a small tablet once daily meets the need. The pituitary, however, produces the hormones that control the adrenal and thyroid glands, and plays a key role in fertility.

Hyperpituitary disorders, sometimes caused by tumors or hyperactive glands, are dealt with by surgery to remove the gland. Sometimes medications such as gonadotropin blocking agents (see Chapter 19) are useful. One more common pituitary problem, though, is growth hormone deficiency. Growth hormone, natural or produced by recombinant DNA techniques, is administered as a replacement. The process does produce growth, but adverse effect risks include hyperglycemia and carpal tunnel syndrome.

The adrenal glands are also crucial for our survival. These small organs (roughly 5 grams each) crowning each kidney produce mineralocorticoids and glucocorticoids. Mineralcorticoids are responsible for maintaining potassium, sodium, and water balance (Porth). Glucocorticoid hormones, mainly cortisol, regulate glucose, protein, and fat metabolism. The table details drugs frequently used for adrenal dysfunction:

### Figure 30: Adrenal dysfunction medications

| Medication | Mechanisms | Potential adverse effects |
|---|---|---|
| Hydrocortisone: equivalent to naturally produced cortisol; used to treat Addison's disease (insufficient natural production of adrenal hormones) | Replacement of natural corticosteroids | Minimal when given in replacement doses; if larger doses are give to treat autoimmune or inflammation, Cushing's disease symptoms can develop* |
| Fludrocortisone—mineralcorticoid used to treat Addison's disease | | Minimal at replacement level doses |

*Cushing's symptoms include: fat deposition on the back ("buffalo hump"), a round "moon" face, muscle weakness, muscle wasting, thin fragile skin, osteoporosis, diabetes, hypokalemia, hypernatremia, susceptibility to infection, and gastric ulcers with bleeding.

## Let's squeeze replacement therapy in

 **Don't forget:** You should be briefly reviewing all of the prior chapters every few days or so, just to carve those memories deeper. If you are already seeing patients or can picture people you know who have some of the disorders we examine in class, great! Linking the content to clinical or actual situations is a brilliant learning strategy.

We will spend the last moments of this lesson discussing hormone replacement therapy (HRT), specifically estrogens and androgens. The table below describes some of the medications used:

### Figure 31: Hormone replacement therapy medications

| Medication | Mechanisms | Potential adverse effects |
|---|---|---|
| Androgens: male hormones Testosterone, Fluoxymesterone | Replacement therapy to treat male hypogonadism (lack of sexual development), breast cancer in women, and wasting due to decreased testosterone levels in patients with AIDS; often abused by athletes to increase muscle mass | Virilization (acne, deepening of voice, baldness, menstrual changes, clitoral enlargement) when taken by females, hepatotoxicity, worsen cholesterol levels, mood changes |
| Estrogens (progestins are often included to counter act the effects of estrogen on the uterus endometrium)—given as replacement therapy to women | Replacement therapy: strengthens bone, reduces cholesterol levels, relief of vasomotor symptoms (hot flashes), prevent urogenital atrophy, decrease risk of colorectal cancer | Nausea, anorexia, increased risk of heart attack, endometrial cancer (unless progestin given with estrogen), breast cancer risk, ovarian cancer risk, dementia risk |

Hormone replacements are most often used in women to lessen the distressing symptoms associated with menopause. Whether or not this is a universally good or harmful practice is, at this moment, uncertain (one of those things to watch in your careers since research is ongoing!) But the bottom line is that HRT may be appropriate for some women when they and their healthcare providers evaluate and weigh potential risks and benefits.

## References

Lehne, R. (2007). *Pharmacology for Nursing Care*, 6th ed. St. Louis: Elsevier.

"National Diabetes Statistics." National Diabetes Information Clearinghouse. Available at *www.diabetes.niddk.nih.gov/dm/pubs/statistics.* Accessed December 17, 2007.

Porth, C. (2004). *Essentials of Pathophysiology*, 6th ed. Philadelphia: Lippincott Williams & Wilkins.

Wilson, B., Shannon, M., Shields, K., and Stang, C. (2007). *Nurse's Drug Guide 2007.* Upper Saddle River, New Jersey: Prentice Hall.

# Chapter 18

# Away we go with antimicrobials

Welcome back! In today's lesson, we will look at mobilizing our defenses against external enemies using antimicrobials. Microbe refers to assorted life forms including bacteria, parasites, and fungus. The jury is still out on viruses: People in the know respectfully disagree whether they are living organisms. The medication term we are most familiar with is antibiotic (or "anti-life"), but what we actually understand this to mean is something lethal to bacteria. Our discussion will honor that common usage and use antimicrobial—perhaps new to some of you—to refer to a broad category with the individual members:

- Antibiotics: effective against bacteria

- Antivirals: used to treat viral infections

- Antifungals: substances effective in fungal diseases

So, why do we care?

Not to belabor the point, but some of us may need to change our mind-set to understand antibiotics are not effective against common colds (viral infections) or issues such as athlete's foot (fungal infection).

**Don't forget:** The entire prescribed amount of the medication MUST BE TAKEN (sorry for shouting) in order to completely eradicate the harmful organism and decrease the chance of the organism developing resistance.

Note there are also drugs used to treat internal (worms, liver flukes, etc.) and external (fleas, lice, scabies) parasites. We won't be discussing these in this lesson since you are not apt to encounter them as frequently as bacterial-, viral-, and fungal-related disorders.

## Battling bacterial infections

There are eukaryocytes (possess cell nuclei), and then there are bacteria. Bacteria are strange organisms in that they are the only life forms that don't possess a true nucleus. These creatures present themselves as cocci (round) or bacilli (elongated rod, may be straight or spiral) shapes and contain a single strand of DNA threaded throughout the cytoplasm. Bacteria are classified based on:

- Appearance: For example, whether cocci (plural form of coccus) appear singly or in clusters or chains.

- Ability to tolerate air: Aerobes can and may need to live in the presence of oxygen; anaerobes do not.

- Presence of cell walls and membranes: Those with a cell wall are gram positive (refers to the ability to turn color in response to gram stain); those with a cell wall and a cell membrane are gram negative.

- Response to antibiotics: Termed susceptible, resistant, or intermediately resistant.

An example will help put it together. The characteristics of one bacterium include gram positive cocci in clusters resistant to the effects of methicillin. The experienced healthcare provider would use this description to indicate methicillin resistant Staphylococcus aureus (MRSA), a particularly tough bacterium responsible for infections that are difficult to vanquish. The Centers for Disease Control and Prevention noted a doubling of hospitalizations related to this bacterium between 1999 and 2005 and urge that it be considered a national health priority (CDC).

Let's look at some of the medications used to treat bacterial infections.

**Don't forget:** Antibiotics are effective only with bacterial infections.

**Figure 32: Bacterial infection medications**

| Medication | Mechanisms | Potential adverse effects |
|---|---|---|
| **Penicillins** (oral, IM, IV)<br>Penicillin G<br>Nafcillin<br>Ampicillin<br>Amoxicillin | Weaken or rupture the bacterial cell wall during growth and reproduction; some are resistant to beta-lactamase produced by particular bacteria; vary in spectrum (range of organisms affected) | Primary adverse reaction is allergy; sometimes life threatening anaphylaxis; diarrhea or GI upset can occur |
| **Cephalosporins**<br>(Oral, IM, IV) Cephalexin, Cefaclor, Cefixime<br>Vancomycin (IV)<br><br>**Glycopeptide** (IV)<br>Vancomycin | Also weaken the cell wall<br><br>Also weaken the cell wall | Most serious side effects for cephalosporins are allergic reactions and GI upset; for vancomycin: ototoxicity (damage to hearing), can cause flushing when administered to rapidly (Red Man's Syndrome—not a true allergy) |
| **Tetracyclines**<br>(Oral, IV, IM)<br>Tetracycline<br>Doxycycline<br>Minocycline | Inhibit bacterial protein synthesis; may also cause alterations in the cytoplasmic membrane | Stains developing teeth, promotes overgrowth of other species (suprainfection) such as yeast, hepatotoxicity, renal toxicity |
| **Aminoglycosides**<br>Gentamycin<br>Tobramycin | Inhibits bacterial protein synthesis resulting in a defective cell membrane | Ototoxicity, nephrotoxicity, blood levels must be monitored |
| **Folic acid antagonist**<br>Sulfamethoxazole and Trimethoprim | Inhibit synthesis of folic acid by bacteria | Hypersensitivity reactions, severe rash (Stevens-Johnson syndrome), hemolytic anemia, kidney damage from crystals in urine |

## Us vs. viral infections

A virus is an infinitesimally tiny parasite that must abide within a cell since it has no intrinsic metabolic capability or activity. It is solely a core of nucleic acid (DNA or RNA) surrounded by a protective coating.

 **Did you know:** There are at least 200 identified viruses able to create disease within humans (Myers).

The virus that causes acquired immunodeficiency syndrome (AIDS) is one of them. Viruses mutate rapidly, which makes them spectacularly adept at developing resistance to medications. This means a detailed discussion of antiviral protocols here will be outdated in weeks to months. So, let's look at a few prototype medications to illustrate basic concepts:

## Figure 33: Antiviral medications

| Medication | Mechanisms | Potential adverse effects |
|---|---|---|
| Acyclovir: used to treat herpes infections (Zovirax®) | Suppresses synthesis of viral DNA | Nausea, vomiting, diarrhea, headache, vertigo |
| Ganciclovir: treatment for cytomegalovirus (CMV) infections (Cytovene®) | Inhibits replication of DNA | Bone marrow suppression, birth defects, nausea, vomiting, confusion, liver dysfunction |
| Amantadine: flu treatment (Symmetrel®) | Prevents viral penetration into host at a cellular level | Dizziness, nervousness, insomnia |
| Zidovudine: HIV treatment (only one drug from four or five subclasses of HIV meds) (Retrovin®) | Suppresses DNA synthesis | Bone marrow suppression, lactic acidosis, nausea, vomiting, diarrhea, insomnia, confusion, myopathy (damage to muscle fibers) |

## The fight against fungal infections

A fungus is a eukaryotic (has a nucleus in each cell) organism that feeds on organic molecules it finds in its environment. A fungal infection is inflammation and tissue destruction caused by fungal infestation. Of the 100,000 identified species, 100 are common in humans and 10 cause disease (Myers). It is fair to say that many fungi are opportunistic and generally do not cause infections if the host is in good health. Opportunistic infections do occur in persons struggling with chronic diseases such as diabetes, AIDS, emphysema, and so on (Merck, Fung). Fungal cells and mammalian cells tend to have a lot of similarities. Substances effective against fungal infections may have significant toxicities for humans. Here are some commonly prescribed antifungal medications.

**Figure 34: Antifungal medications**

| Medication | Mechanisms | Potential adverse effects |
|---|---|---|
| Amphotericin B (IV) | Increases permeability of fungal cell membrane by binding to ergosterol (a component of the fungal cell membrane) | Infusion reactions (fever, chills, headache, nausea), nephrotoxicity, hypokalemia, bone marrow suppression |
| Itraconazole (Oral, IV) (Sporanox®) | Inhibits fungal cell membrane formation by blocking synthesis of ergosterol | Nausea, vomiting, diarrhea, headache, cardiac toxicity, hepatotoxicity |
| Fluconazole (Diflucan®) | Inhibits fungal cell membrane formation by blocking synthesis of ergosterol | Nausea, headache, rash, abdominal pain |

## Two minutes on tuberculosis

Our last topic in this lesson is tuberculosis (TB). By rights, we should have considered it in the bacterial infection section because the causative agent, mycobacterium tuberculosis, is a bacterium. This is an unusual situation. The disease has been around forever, waxes and wanes, and currently is reemerging as a potent threat to world health. In 2006, the World Health Organization reported there were 9 million new cases and 2 million deaths worldwide in 2004. Though 80% of all new cases develop in people living in sub-Saharan Africa or Asia, the entire world is at risk due to the limitless mobility of the population.

**Did you know:** Because of the emergence of drug resistant strains (due in large part to inadequately or incompletely treated patients) all tuberculosis cases should be treated with at least three or four medications, and there are now some strains that don't respond well to any medication.

Let's look at some TB medications:

### Figure 35: Tuberculosis medications

| Medication | Mechanisms | Potential adverse effects |
| --- | --- | --- |
| Isoniazid (Oral) (Nydrazid®) | Kills bacteria, but exact mechanism unknown possibly by disruption of the bacterial cell wall | Peripheral neuropathy, hepatotoxicity, nausea, vomiting |
| Rifampin (Oral) (Rifadin®) | Suppresses RNA synthesis | Hepatotoxicity, stains all body fluids red/orange, rash, nausea, vomiting; Optic neuritis, allergic reactions, GI upset |
| Ethambutol (Oral) (Myambutol®) | Suppresses bacterial reproduction and interferes with RNA synthesis | Hepatotoxicity, joint aches, nausea, vomiting |
| Pyrazinamide (Oral) | Kills bacteria, but exact mechanism unknown | Hepatotoxicity, joint aches, nausea, vomiting |

Typically, patients must take their antitubercular medications for up to a year to ensure complete treatment. That is a long time to endure unpleasant side effects that, coupled with cost, account for limited patient compliance and the development of resistant strains.

We just scratched the surface of billions and billions of antimicrobial drugs. Okay, maybe that was just a smidge of hyperbole there, but there are tons! Don't be overwhelmed.

### Don't forget:

1.  Learn the general characteristics of each type (antiviral, antifungal, etc.)

2.  Study categories (penicillins, for example) vs. drug by drug

3.  Become familiar with unique features of particular medications (stained body fluids with rifampin, for example)

# References

"Bacteria: Basic Facts." The Merck Manual of Diagnosis and Therapy. Available at *www.microbiologybytes.com/iandi/3a.html*. Accessed December 18, 2007.

"Hospitalizations and Deaths Caused by Methicillin-Resistant Staphylococcus aureus, United States, 1999–2005." Centers for Disease Control and Prevention. Available at *www.cdc.gov/eid/content/13/12/1840.htm*. Accessed December 18, 2007.

"Introduction: Fungi." The Merck Manuals Online Medical Library. Available at *www.merck.com/mmpe/sec14/ch180/ch180a.html?qt=fungal% 20infections&alt=sh*. Accessed December 18, 2007.

"Global Tuberculosis Control." World Health Organization Report, 2006. Available at *www.who.int/tb/publications/global_report/2006/pdf/full_report.pdf*. Accessed December 18, 2007.

Lehne, R. (2007). *Pharmacology for Nursing Care*, 6th ed. St. Louis: Elsevier.

Myers, T. (ed) (2006). *Mosby's Dictionary of Medicine, Nursing & Health Professions*, 7th ed. St. Louis, Missouri. Elsevier.

Porth, C. (2004). *Essentials of Pathophysiology*, 6th ed. Philadelphia: Lippincott Williams & Wilkins.

Wilson, B., Shannon, M., Shields, K., and Stang, C. (2007). *Nurse's Drug Guide 2007*. Upper Saddle River, New Jersey: Prentice Hall.

# Chapter 19

# A little time with antineoplastic medications

This lesson will have us consider the medications used to treat cancer. Because this is such a specialized area and is rapidly changing, our conversation will be limited to a review of general cancer disease concepts and an introduction of the broad categories of antineoplastic medications.

## Considering cancers

Let's be precise for a minute: All cancers are neoplasms, but not all neoplasms are necessarily cancers. For example, the harmless raised mole on your cheek or the extra skin hanging off of grandpa's neck are both neoplasms—but not cancers. That being said, we are referring to anticancer effects when we talk about antineoplastic medications. Keep your dictionary handy because each cancer's name gives a clue. For example, leuk (white blood cells) emia (blood) refers to abnormal amounts and types of white blood cells. Likewise, sarc (muscle) oma (tumor) indicates a tumor in muscles.

Cancer is not a rare phenomenon. The American Cancer Society (ACS) estimated there would be 1,339,790 new cases of cancer and 564,830 deaths in 2006 (ACS, 2006).

**Did you know:** The ACS also estimates that approximately half of all American men and one-third of American women will develop some form (ranging from relatively harmless to lethal) of cancer in their lifetime! It's easy to see why there is such an extraordinary interest in new and more effective cancer treatments.

What is cancer? Cancer cells don't undergo normal proliferation and differentiation and fail to "play nice" with other cells. The dangerous ones share a cluster of characteristics:

- They are undifferentiated and bear little resemblance to the normal tissue from which they arose

- They grow and infiltrate or destroy surrounding tissue

- Growth rates are variable, with the least differentiated growing at the fastest rate

- Cells can break off from primary sites and migrate to distant locations through the blood or lymph circulation

- Cancers can cause nonspecific or generalized effects such as anemia, weight loss, and weakness

- Cancers frequently cause death because of their uncontrolled growth (Porth)

The goal of antineoplastic medications, or chemotherapy, is to kill the cancer without killing the patient. This is a huge challenge due to the significant anatomic and physiologic characteristics that are common to both normal host cells and malignant cancer tissue. Remember, as always, that up-to-the-moment information is not likely to be found in books. You will find the latest information on the Internet:

**Click:** The U.S. Food and Drug Administration Center for Drug Evaluation and Research's oncology tools page is a great starting point: *www.fda.gov/cder/cancer/approved.htm*

**Click:** Select the name of a particular drug, and you will find comprehensive information on MedlinePlus that you can share with your patients using lay language rather than professional terminology: *www.nlm.nih.gov/medlineplus/druginfo/drug_Aa.html*

**Click:** Cancer Care Ontario is another comprehensive site that provides practical information for both consumers and healthcare providers: *www.cancercare.on.ca/index_drugFormularymonographs.htm*

## Clustering cancer medications

Let's consider examples of the broad categories used to cluster cancer medication. Keep in mind that many anticancer medications are potentially dangerous to even handle, and most are only administered by a nurse that has undergone specialized instruction. The following tables provide a general overview:

Alkylating drugs alter DNA bonds in fast-growing cells.

### Figure 36: Alkylating medications

| Medication | Mechanisms | Potential adverse effects |
|---|---|---|
| Cyclophosamide (Cytoxan®): a nitrogen mustard type for Hodgkin's and non-Hodgkin's lymphomas, multiple myeloma, and some solid tumors of head, neck, ovary, and breast

Carmustine (BCNU®): a nitrosourea type used for brain tumors, lymphomas, multiple myeloma, melanoma, and cancers of stomach, colon, and rectum

Cisplatin (Platinol®): a platinum-containing drug used for testicular, ovarian, and bladder cancers | These substances kill cells by using an alkyl group to form a covalent bond between two guanine molecules in DNA | Injure all cells that grow rapidly and result in low white blood cells (neutropenia), low platelets (thrombocytopenia), low red blood cells (anemia), hair loss, ulcerations of GI mucous membranes, nausea, vomiting; all are vesicants (damage tissues on contact) and must be carefully administered by IV into large blood vessels; cancers can develop resistance to these medications |

Antimetabolic drugs resemble natural substances and disrupt metabolism. They are used to treat cancer and some autoimmune disorders.

### Figure 37: Antimetabolic medications

| Medication | Mechanisms | Potential adverse effects |
|---|---|---|
| Methotrexate (Amethopterin®): kills cells by inhibiting DNA synthesis, folic acid analog; used to treat lymphomas, leukemias, sarcomas, also rheumatoid arthritis and psoriasis<br><br>Cytarabine (ARA-C): a pyrimidine analog used to treat leukemias<br><br>Mercaptopurine (Purinethol®): a purine analog used for leukemias | These medications are either folic acid analogs (imitate, but have different properties), purine (one class of DNA and RNA nitrogen bases) analogs, or pyrimidine (the other class of DNA and RNA nitrogen bases) analogs; chemical reactions are inhibited when these analogs 'fool' cells; causes cell death | Bone suppression resulting in neutropenia, thrombocytopenia, anemia; oral and GI ulcerations |

Antiandrogen drugs are primarily used to treat prostate cancer in men by modifying male hormone production or response to male hormones.

### Figure 38: Antiandrogen medications

| Medication | Mechanisms | Potential adverse effects |
|---|---|---|
| Leuprolide (Lupron®) (gonadotropin releasing hormone agonist): used for prostate cancer and emdometriosis<br><br>Flutamide (Eulexin®) (androgen receptor blocker): used for prostate cancer<br><br>Abarelix (Plenaxis®) (gonadotropin releasing hormone antagonist): used for advanced prostate cancer | Gonadotropin-releasing hormone agonist; inhibits the production of androgens by the testes<br><br>Gonadotropin-releasing hormone antagonist; inhibits the production of androgens by the testes by inhibiting the pituitary gland<br><br>Androgen (male hormone) receptor blockers; prevents the effect of androgens | Hot flashes, impotence, loss of libido (sexual interest and drive), increased risk of bone fractures, nausea vomiting, diarrhea, gynecomastia or breast enlargement (with androgen blockers), allergic reactions |

Antiestrogen drugs are primarily used for breast cancer.

### Figure 39: Antiestrogen medications

| Medication | Mechanisms | Potential adverse effects |
|---|---|---|
| Fulvestrant (Faslodex®) Tamoxifen (Nolvedex®) Toremifene (Fareston®) | Block estrogen receptors; works only for breast cancers whose growth is stimulated by estrogen | Hot flashes, fluid retention, vaginal discharge, vomiting, irregular menstruation, and endometrial cancer |

Antibiotic drugs are used only for cancer and never to treat infections.

### Figure 40: Antibiotic medications

| Medication | Mechanisms | Potential adverse effects |
|---|---|---|
| Doxorubicin (Adriamycin®): an anthracycline type used for many types of cancers Daunorubicin (Cerubidine®) (daunomycin): very similar to doxorubicin Dactinomycin (Actinomycin-D®): a nonanthracycline used for Wilms' tumor, sarcomas, testicular cancer, choriocarcinomas | Despite their name, they are used only to treat cancer and never to treat infections. They kill cancers by altering the shape of DNA | All anthracylcines can cause heart damage, all cause severe bone marrow depression; the nonanthracyclines do not damage the heart but can cause severe bone marrow depression and ulcerations of the mouth and GI tract; other side effects for both classes may include nausea, vomiting, hair loss |

Here are some examples of antimitotic drugs:

**Figure 41: Antimitotic medications**

| Medication | Mechanisms | Potential adverse effects |
|---|---|---|
| Vincristine (Oncovin®): used for lymphomas, sarcomas, leukemias, Wilms' tumor, breast cancer, bladder cancer<br><br>Paclitaxel (Taxol®): used for ovarian cancer, certain types of lung cancer, breast cancer | These all act in the M phase of mitosis to prevent cell division | Peripheral neuropathy, vesicant, hair loss, bone marrow suppression with paclitaxel but not vincristine |

Finally, here are a few other cancer drugs:

**Figure 42: A few other cancer medications**

| Medication | Mechanisms | Potential adverse effects |
|---|---|---|
| Interferon Alfa 2a and 2b: both used to treat leukemias and Kaposi's sarcoma Interleukin-2: used to treat melanoma and renal cancer | Immunostimulants: complete action still unclear, but these are thought to increase the patient immune response and decrease proliferation of cancer cells | Potential adverse effects Fever, chills, fatigue, anorexia, nausea, vomiting, interleukin-2 has a 4% mortality rate |
| **Targeted drugs** Cetuximab (Erbitux®): an antibody used for particular colorectal cancers Rituximab (Rituxan®): an antibody used for B-cell non-Hodgkin's lymphoma Imatinib (Gleevec®): a small molecule used for myeloid leukemia and GI stromal tumors | Designed to bind and inhibit specific molecules that promote tumor growth | Varies with particular drug but many cause rash, fever and chills, bone marrow depression, nausea, and diarrhea |

# Before the bell rings . . .

Let's summarize this lesson: We began by considering terminology, examining cancer characteristics, and recognizing the goal of chemotherapy. We also learned that chemotherapy administration is a pretty intense discipline beyond the scope of most nurses unless they've undergone additional study and training.

The key things to remember are:

- We need to learn the general framework and important concepts from texts and augment that with timely information searches of reputable online sources.

- All chemotherapies have toxicities due to their interaction with physiologic mechanisms common to both cancerous and normal tissue.

- Because antineoplastic drugs often target fast-growing cancer cells, they also run the risk of causing side effects in fast growing normal tissues, such as bone marrow, hair, and mucous membranes. Specific adverse reactions include bone marrow suppression, alopecia, and GI toxicity.

- Some potential side effects are related to the mechanism of action. Hormonal modifiers, for example, alter the effect of either male or female hormones.

You are nearly through with Part 3! Don't fade away just yet. Too much information, you say? You need something for a headache? Hold that thought: nonsteroidal anti-inflammatories and acetaminophen are next!

## References

"Approved Oncology Drugs." U.S. Food and Drug Administration, Oncology Tools. Available at *www.fda.gov/cder/cancer/approved.htm*. Accessed December 16, 2007.

Lehne, R. (2007). *Pharmacology for Nursing Care*, 6th ed. St. Louis: Elsevier.

Porth, C. (2004). *Essentials of Pathophysiology*, 6th ed. Philadelphia: Lippincott Williams & Wilkins.

Springhouse (2003). *Professional Guide to Pathophysiology*. Philadelphia: Lippincott Williams & Wilkins.

Venes, D. and Thomas, C. (eds) (2001). *Taber's Cylcopedic Medical Dictionary*. Philadelphia: F.A. Davis Company.

Wilson, B., Shannon, M., Shields, K., and Stang, C. (2007). *Nurse's Drug Guide 2007*. Upper Saddle River, New Jersey: Prentice Hall.

# Chapter 20

# Anti-inflammatory and immune system modifiers 101

Welcome back! We are going to look at medications that influence our immune response in this class. In addition, we will examine a very common drug that fits with no other category we have considered before and won't fit with any in our future lessons. Let's get started.

There is a class of medications called glucocorticoids (we touched on them briefly in Chapter 15). These mimic the effects of substances produced by our own adrenal glands. The naturally produced hormones maintain the integrity of blood vessel walls, maintain blood pressure and blood sugar levels during times of stress, play a huge role in metabolism regulation, reduce inflammation from injury, and, overall, keep us functioning. We can't survive without them. The glucocorticoid medications are primarily given to reduce excessive inflammatory responses (pain, swelling, itching, heat, leakage of fluid from blood vessels, collections of leukocytes, release of proteases and histamine) associated with disease. Long-term use of these medications cause complications such as altered fluid balance, altered fat storage, hyperglycemia (elevated blood sugar), osteoporosis, decreased immune response (leaving the patient open to opportunistic infections), skin changes, and fungal infections among others.

## Speaking about NSAIDs

Our first category is the nonsteroidal anti-inflammatory drugs (NSAIDs). The name is supremely straightforward and accurate.

Imagine you are on the way to pharmacology class. You are silently perusing your cardiovascular medication flash cards while sitting at a stop light, when all of a sudden, WHAAAMMM!—a car crunches into the back of yours! Picture yourself slowly inventorying your body and testing for injury; everything seems okay. After you and the other driver exchange insurance information, you continue on your way.

The next day, your neck aches, the muscles are tight, and you have difficulty turning your head. You mosey on to the urgent care facility where they determine everything is fine, but the doctor suggests ibuprofen to relieve your discomfort. Imagine that you pop a couple of tablets as she suggested, and you are comfortable within 45 minutes. What happened?

This class of drugs is very effective for mild to moderate pain, and it all began with aspirin. There is a ton of anecdotal history about people chewing on willow bark and other natural substances that contain salicylates—all of it shrouded in the misty confusion of myth and history.

 **Did you know:** One thing is certain: Aspirin was first marketed by Bayer (thanks to the work of a German chemist named Felix Hoffmann) in 1899 and has been used pretty steadily ever since.

Over time, people noticed that aspirin users developed ulcers and gastrointestinal bleeding. Also, researchers found a connection between Reye's syndrome (a combination of encephalopathy and fatty infiltration of organs) and aspirin use in children with viral illnesses. Aspirin is the original NSAID. All of the others came as an effort to develop more effective drugs with fewer side effects. The most commonly used NSAIDs (of the 25-plus available) are listed in the following table.

But before we get there, let's talk quickly about an enzyme called cyclooxygenase (COX), which comes in two forms.

- COX1 contributes toward protecting our gastric mucosa, inhibiting bleeding, and aids renal function. Inhibiting this enzyme promotes ulcer formation, prolongs bleeding times, and can leave the kidney open to damage.

- COX2 contributes toward development of pain, inflammation, and fever.

All the medications listed below inhibit COX1 and COX2, except for the selective COX2 agent, celecoxib. They decrease our natural body's responses that give rise to inflammation.

### Figure 43: Common NSAIDs

| Medication | Mechanisms | Potential adverse effects |
|---|---|---|
| Aspirin (Bayer®) | Inhibits COX 1 & 2; given for arthritis, moderate pain, fever | GI bleeding due to ulceration, prolonged bleeding due to decreased platelet aggregation, hypersensitivity reactions |
| Ibuprofen (Advil®) | Inhibits COX 1 & 2; given for arthritis, moderate pain, fever, dysmenorrhea (pain during menstruation), bursitis/tendonitis | Less gastric bleeding than aspirin but still possible; may increase risk of stroke and heart attack |
| Naproxen (Naprosyn®) | Inhibits COX 1 & 2; given for arthritis, moderate pain, fever, dysmenorrhea, bursitis/tendonitis | Generally well tolerated; can cause GI upset; decreased renal function; may increase risk of stroke and heart attack |
| Indomethacin (Indocin®) | Inhibits COX 1 & 2; given for arthritis, moderate pain, bursitis/tendonitis | Severe headache, dizziness, confusion, nausea, vomiting, GI bleeding; may increase risk of stroke and heart attack |
| Celecoxib (Celebrex®) | Inhibits COX2; given for arthritis, moderate pain, dysmenorrhea | Still a risk of GI bleeding despite no action on COX1; associated with increase risk of adverse cardiovascular events, including myocardial infarction |

**Click:** This page at MedicineNet.com is an impressive NSAID information source you can share with patients: *www.medicinenet.com/nonsteroidal_ antiinflammatory_drugs/article.htm*

## More potent meds: Immunosuppressants

There are other much more potent drugs that inhibit our body's responses and are used to prevent organ rejection after transplantation surgery.

These drugs have specific applications. Here are some of the more common ones:

## Figure 44: Common immunosuppressants

| Medication | Mechanisms | Potential adverse effects |
|---|---|---|
| Cyclosporine: Calcineurin inhibitor (Sandimmune®) | Inhibits interleukin-2 (IL2) and interferon gamma production; used to prevent organ rejection and to treat autoimmune diseases such as rheumatoid arthritis and psoriasis; given orally or IV | Nephrotoxicity (toxic to kidney), hepatotoxicity (toxic to liver), lymphoma, anaphylaxis, diarrhea, vomiting, hypertension, hyperkalemia, gingival hyperplasia (overgrowth of gums); must monitor drug levels and kidney function |
| Tacrolimus: Calcineurin inhibitor (Prograf®) | More effective than cyclosporine, but a similar mechanism | More toxic than cyclosporine, nephrotoxicity most common; diarrhea, vomiting, hypertension, hyperkalemia |
| Muromonab-CD3: Monoclonal antibody (OrthocloneOKT®) | Binds to IL2 receptors on white blood cells; given post-transplant to prevent organ rejection | Fever, chills, dyspnea, chest pain, nausea, vomiting, anaphylaxis, infection |
| Mycophenolate mofetil (CellCept®) | Inhibits T lympho sites | Tremor, headache, insomnia, hyptertension, constipation/diarrhea, renal impairment, anemia, infection |

## Earn an 'A' in acetaminophen

The last medication we'll be discussing in this lesson seems vaguely related to NSAIDS but in reality is entirely different. Tylenol®, the original brand name for acetaminophen, was introduced in 1955 as a prescribed alternative to aspirin. In those days, as mentioned above, researchers had begun to note a link between Reye's syndrome and aspirin use. Consumers were eager for an alternative. Though we think of it as relatively benign, it is interesting to note acetaminophen-associated liver failure is the second most common reason for liver transplants in the United States (Farrell).

| Figure 45: Acetaminophen | | |
| --- | --- | --- |
| **Medication** | **Mechanisms** | **Potential adverse effects** |
| Acetaminophen (Tylenol®) | Inhibits prostaglandins in the CNS; given for fever and mild to moderate pain | Rare at therapeutic doses; overdose can cause liver failure due to a toxic metabolite; should not be used by persons with liver disease or who drink alcoholic beverages regularly |

The last topic we'll cover in Part 3 is nutrition. Take a break, grab a cheese-burger, er, an apple, and we'll get going.

## References

Andermann, A. (1996) "Physicians, Fads, and Pharmaceuticals: A History of Aspirin." Available at *www.medicine.mcgill.ca/mjm/v02n02/aspirin.html.* Accessed December 10, 2007.

Farrell, S. (2007) "Toxicity, Acetaminophen." EMedicine. Available at *www.emedicine.com/emerg/topic819.htm.* Accessed December 10, 2007.

Lehne, R. (2007). *Pharmacology for Nursing Care,* 6th ed. St. Louis: Elsevier. "NINDS Reye's Syndrome Information Page." National Institute of Neurological Disorders and Stroke. Available at *www.ninds.nih.gov/disorders/ reyes_syndrome/reyes_syndrome.htm.* Accessed December 10, 2007.

Porth, C. (2004). *Essentials of Pathophysiology,* 6th ed. Philadelphia: Lippincott Williams & Wilkins.

Springhouse (2003). *Professional Guide to Pathophysiology.* Philadelphia: Lippincott Williams & Wilkins.

Teague, K. (2000). "The history of Tylenol." Available at *www.auburn.edu/ ~teagukl/tyhist.htm.* Accessed December 10, 2007.

Venes, D. and Thomas, C. (eds) (2001). *Taber's Cylcopedic Medical Dictionary.* Philadelphia: F.A. Davis Company.

Wilson, B., Shannon, M., Shields, K., and Stang, C. (2007). *Nurse's Drug Guide 2007.* Upper Saddle River, New Jersey: Prentice Hall.

# Chapter 21

# We live longer if we take vitamins, right?

What is the truth about vitamin C? Does it help cure colds? What about vitamin E preventing cancer or beta-carotene (vitamin A precursor) preventing heart attacks? We know higher dietary intakes of folate and B6 may reduce risk of colorectal cancer in women (Zhang, et al.), for example. We also know that the majority of adults—52%—take at least one vitamin supplement regularly (Radimer, et al.). But what happens if you don't take enough of these things? Or what if you take too much? And what role do minerals play? There are a lot of questions here. Let's begin to examine the answers.

## A vitamin a day . . .

Vitamins are a group of organic compounds that catalyze (permit or speed up reactions without entering into the reaction itself) assorted chemical reactions in our bodies. Generally speaking, vitamins cannot be synthesized in the body. A substance cannot be considered a vitamin unless a deficiency of that substance causes disease (Porth, Myers). Vitamins are either fat soluble (A, D, E, and K) or water soluble (C, and the eight B-complex vitamins: thiamine, riboflavin, niacin, pyridoxine, pantothenic acid, B12, folic acid, and biotin). All vitamins are essential for good health.

Can we maintain good health on poor diets, or if we skip meals, as long as we take vitamins? No. Vitamins are just one component of a balanced diet that also includes sufficient carbohydrates, protein, fats, fiber, and water.

The standard is to ensure intake sufficient to meet the recommended dietary allowance established by the Food and Nutrition Board of the Institute of Medicine of the National Academy of Sciences (Lehne).

The following table of vitamins identifies purpose, uses, and adverse effects:

### Figure 46: Vitamins

| Vitamin | Mechanisms | Potential adverse effects |
|---|---|---|
| Vitamin A | Essential for night vision; deficiency can cause blindness; no evidence that supplementation prevents heart disease or cancer | Toxic at high doses; liver injury, bone disorders; can cause birth defects (teratogenic) |
| Thiamine (B1) | Deficiency can cause beriberi (neurologic and motor deficits); alcoholics can develop deficiency-related dementia (Wernicke-Korsakoff syndrome) | None |
| Riboflavin (B2) | Deficiency produces stomatitis (inflammation of mouth), glossitis (inflammation of tongue), dermatitis (inflammation of skin); can help prevent migraines | None |
| Pyridoxine (B6) | Deficiency exhibits dermatitis, anemia, depression, confusion, peripheral neuritis, seizures; deficiency common in alcoholics | Very large doses can produce ataxia (motor disturbances) and numbness of the hands and feet |
| Folic Acid (B9) | Functions as a coenzyme with B12 and C in protein metabolism; deficiency causes glossitis, stomatitis, GI lesions, neural birth defects | None |
| Cyanocobalamin (B12) | Deficiency causes anemia and neurological damage | None |
| Biotin | Essential for carbohydrate and fat metabolism; deficiency extremely rare since it is found in a wide range of foods | None |
| Vitamin C | Participant in many biochemical reactions; required for collagen synthesis; deficiency causes scurvy (bleeding gums, loose teeth, bruising, faulty bone development); high doses have not been proven to be effective to treat or prevent any disorder from colds to cancer | Nausea, abdominal cramps, diarrhea |
| Vitamin D | Regulates calcium and phosphorous metabolism; deficiency in children causes rickets, osteomalacia in adults—both result in frail deformed bones | Symptoms related to hypercalcemia (anorexia, confusion, abdominal pain, muscle pain, coma, shock, death) |
| Vitamin E | No clearly established nutritional role defined; perhaps maintains health by acting as an antioxidant of lipids; supplementation may reduce risk of colds and protect against Alzheimer's | Bleeding; may accelerate cancer progression |
| Vitamin K | Required for synthesis of four clotting factors; deficiency produces severe bleeding; it is used to reverse warfarin overdose (primary clinical use) | IV and IM administration can cause anaphylaxis; subcutaneous route preferred |

## Cracking the mystery of minerals

Minerals are involved in many processes. Iron, for example is a component of hemoglobin. Calcium, magnesium, sodium, and potassium are all involved in nerve impulse transmission and muscle contraction.

 **Did you know:** Some minerals are macrominerals and are present in large quantities: calcium, phosphorous, sodium, chloride, potassium, magnesium, and sulfur. Others are present only in minute amounts and are termed trace minerals: iron, manganese, copper, iodine, zinc, cobalt, fluorine, and selenium (Porth).

Typically, daily mineral requirements are met by dietary intake if a wide variety of food is consumed. Too much of these substances, however, can cause harm. For example, women's multivitamins contain iron to replace stores lost due to menstruation. Men's vitamins do not. Without regular iron loss, supplementation can cause iron overload (known as hemochromatosis). It can also develop and produce liver injury, cause skin pigmentation changes, diabetes, and cardiac failure (Myers). Selenium gives us another example. It is essential for the normal functioning of the immune system and thyroid, but oversupplementation gives rise to selenosis, a condition characterized by gastrointestinal upsets, hair loss, white blotchy nails, and nerve damage.

So in summary, the answer seems to be to ensure an adequate dietary intake of vitamins and minerals while avoiding excess supplementation.

This is a short lesson because of limited reliable information. Despite a variety of anecdotal reports, there doesn't seem to be any research that clearly supports large nutrient doses targeted to improve or prevent particular diseases. It is also reasonable to not expect much research investigating the efficacy of vitamins. The heavy hitters, as far as research dollars go, are the pharmaceutical companies who do need to make a return on invested resources to ensure survival by creating new products. There are not a lot of funding sources for investigations looking at new uses for common substances or generic medications.

You've made it through Part 3! Let's move on and discover how we can put this information to use in a successful and safe nursing career.

# References

"Dietary supplements: Using vitamin and mineral supplements wisely." MayoClinic.com. Available at *www.mayoclinic.com/print/supplements/NU00198/ METHOD=print*. Accessed December 11, 2007.

Lehne, R. (2007). *Pharmacology for Nursing Care*, 6th ed. St. Louis: Elsevier.

Myers, T. (ed) (2006). *Mosby's Dictionary of Medicine, Nursing & Health Professions*, 7th ed. St. Louis: Elsevier.

Porth, C. (2004). *Essentials of Pathophysiology*, 6th ed. Philadelphia: Lippincott Williams & Wilkins.

Radimer, K., Bindewald, B., Hughes, J., Ervin, B., Swanson, C., and Picciano, M. (2004). "Dietary supplement use by US adults: Data from the national health and nutrition examination survey, 1999-2000." *American Journal of Epidemiology* 160(4): 339-349.

"Selenium." HealthLink: Medical College of Wisconsin. Available at *http:// healthlink.mcw.edu/article/964647329.html*. Accessed December 11, 2007.

Zhang, S., Moore, S., Lin, S., Cook, N., Manson, J., Lee, I., and Buring, J. (2006). "Folate, vitamin B6, multivitamin supplements, and colorectal cancer risk in women." *American Journal of Epidemiology* 183(2): 108-115.

# Part Four

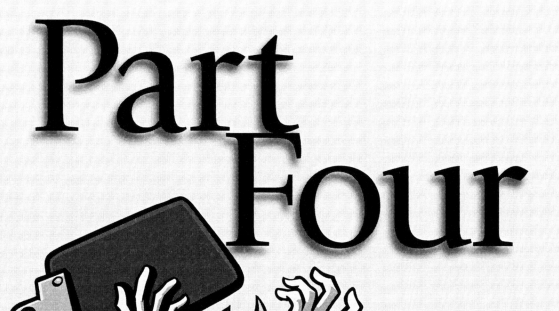

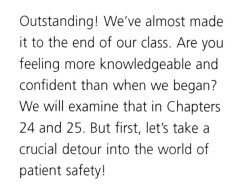

Outstanding! We've almost made it to the end of our class. Are you feeling more knowledgeable and confident than when we began? We will examine that in Chapters 24 and 25. But first, let's take a crucial detour into the world of patient safety!

# Chapter 22

# Avoiding dangerous medication errors

## Real people really get hurt!

In the previous chapters, you learned about the key areas in the selection and administration of medications. These are important skills because we use them every day. A typical hospital patient will receive at least 10 medication doses every day. So, what's your guess? Do we get it right most of the time?

In reality—no, we don't.

A hospital patient can be subject to about one medication error for every day they are in the hospital—and that does not include late or missed doses. That doesn't seem to be very good, but is anyone really getting hurt? YES! There are more than 1,200,000 (that's 1.2 *million*!) adverse drug events every year in hospitals and long-term care facilities. Not only does this result in preventable deaths and a reduction in care and treatment, it also costs more than $3.5 billion every year. (Aspden, et al.)

Preventing medication errors is vitally important because real people— your patients, their families, your family, your friends, and perhaps even you—get hurt.

This chapter focuses on what we all need to do every day to prevent medication errors. So pay attention, learn some easy-to-use error reduction tools, and move to the head of the class!

## It can happen to anyone . . .

This medication error happened at a world-famous hospital to the two newborn children of a famous actor.

### A medication miscue

"On November 18, three patients who were receiving intravenous medications as part of their treatment had their IV catheters flushed with a solution containing a higher concentration of heparin (a medication used to keep IV catheters from clotting) than normal protocol. As a result of a preventable error, the patients' IV catheters were *flushed with heparin from vials containing a concentration of 10,000 units per milliliter instead of from vials containing a concentration of 10 units per milliliter.*"

"The error was identified by Cedars-Sinai staff, who immediately performed blood tests on the patients to measure blood clotting function. … Two patients were given protamine sulfate, a drug that reverses the effects of heparin and helps restore blood clotting function to normal. Additional medical tests and clinical evaluation conducted on the two patients indicated no adverse effects from the higher concentration of heparin or from the temporary abnormal clotting function. Doctors continue to monitor the patients."

"I want to extend my deepest apologies to the families who were affected by this situation, and we will continue to work with them on any concerns or questions they may have. *This was a preventable error, involving a failure to follow our standard policies and procedures, and there is no excuse for that to occur at Cedars-Sinai.* Although it appears at this point that there was no harm to any patient, we take this situation very seriously. We are conducting a comprehensive investigation, cooperating fully with the Los Angeles County Department of Health Services, and will take all necessary steps to ensure that this never happens here again."

—*Statement of Michael L. Langberg, MD, Chief Medical Officer, Cedars-Sinai Medical Center, November 20, 2007 (bolding, italics added for effect)*

## Statistics about medication errors
**Did you know:**

- In hospitals, there are estimated to be more than 400,000 preventable adverse drug events (ADEs) every year

- Adverse dug events cost hospitals about $3.5 billion dollars every year

- In long-term care, there are estimated to be more than 800,000 preventable ADEs every year

- Medication administration errors happen in about 11% of the administrations—excluding "wrong time" errors

- On average, a hospital patient is subject to at least one medication error per day (Aspden, et al.)

# A quick medication error quiz

Are these medication errors?
Yes or no?

1. We administer aspirin 81mg PRN instead of ibuprofen.

2. We forget to record the requested dose change order in the chart that was given to us verbally by the physician.

3. We hang the right IV bag—but on the wrong patient.

4. We pull the medications out of the automatic dispensing system for two patients and put them in our pocket so we don't have to walk back down the hall. They get mixed up.

5. Two syringes are on the cart. We pick up the wrong one and administer a powerful nerve block instead of an epidural. The patient arrests.

6. Things are so busy we forget to give Mrs. Smith her 2:00 dose.

Hopefully, you answered "yes" to each of the questions. Each one is an example of a medication error.

# Let's break down medication errors

If we want to prevent medication errors, we first need to understand a little about why human errors occur. First, errors occur because we are human—yes, we are not perfect. If you think about your day, you have probably made quite a few errors today. Maybe you spilled your soda at lunch, maybe you backed out of the parking spot without looking, or perhaps you forgot your badge or keys.

Everyone makes errors. Astronauts, pilots, surgeons, physicians, nurses, and even hospital administrators make errors. That's an important starting point, but the real issue is in preventing harm. We all chose to work in healthcare rather than at a large retail store. Unlike a job in retail, in healthcare, the decisions and actions you take everyday directly influence the health, comfort, and even the very life of those with whom you deal. That is why working in healthcare can be so rewarding, but it is also why we need to be absolutely vigilant to prevent harm by preventing errors that can affect our patients, our coworkers, and ourselves.

 **Watch out:** A typical human error might be to transpose two numbers. We think 51 when the number really is 15.

Retail: If we work in retail, and our job is to price pencils, we might make the error of pricing a 15-cent pencil for 51 cents. Is there harm? Well it certainly is a mistake, and our boss might be mad at us, but no one will die.

Healthcare: What if we make the same mistake in selecting a medication dose and give our patient 51 mgs instead of 15 mgs, or we transpose two digits in the patient identifier? Is there the potential for harm? Absolutely.

 **Don't forget:** What appears to be just "normal human errors" can be life threatening in healthcare, and we must be focused on preventing them all the time—every day.

### People + systems + equipment = errors
To have a highly reliable medication process, we need three things to all work well together.

1.  The people (that's us)

2.  The systems (that's the policies, procedures, and methods that we get trained on)

3.  The equipment (that's the computers, the pumps, the automatic dis-
    pensing equipment, etc.)

All of these parts, working together, prevent harm to our patients that might
come from a medication error.

There are two simple but powerful mental models that help us understand
the foundations of why errors happen. These two models are called the
Swiss Cheese Barrier Model and GEMS.

## The Swiss Cheese Model

James Reason, a British psychologist, developed a powerful model to help
us understand why errors happen in complex systems such as medication
administration. Figure 47 shows the three key parts of the model. To simplify this very powerful model, let's look at those three parts.

First, there are triggers, those things that start the snowball of an error happening. These triggers could be a human error ("oops, I forgot to check"),
an equipment failure ("the PCA pump broke") or an external event ("snow
storm, hurricane, power failure"). These are on the left side of the figure.

Second, we are committed to the safety of our patients and coworkers, so
we design protections, or barriers, to stop errors before they result in harm.
These have to catch that snowball of an error and keep it from getting bigger and hurting someone. What barriers do we put into place to keep errors
from growing into harm? How about training? That's a good barrier. So are
supervision, good procedures, well-designed equipment, good lighting, and
good error reduction tools.

The third part of the Swiss Cheese Model is on the right hand side of the
figure. It is a significant event or a serious medication error that results in
harm. That's what we want to prevent.

So if the snowball of an error starts rolling down the hill, how many of the
barriers need to fail to result in a medication error? If all the barriers have
a hole in them, any error trigger will go right through each barrier and ultimately reach the patient and likely cause harm.

So the next question is "How many successful barriers does it take to stop an
error from causing harm?" Here is where you become so powerful: If only

one of the barriers works, if you use good technique and use error reduction tools effectively, you can be the barrier that stops an error from reaching a patient or causing harm.

 **Don't forget:** It takes only one effective barrier to stop a medication error!

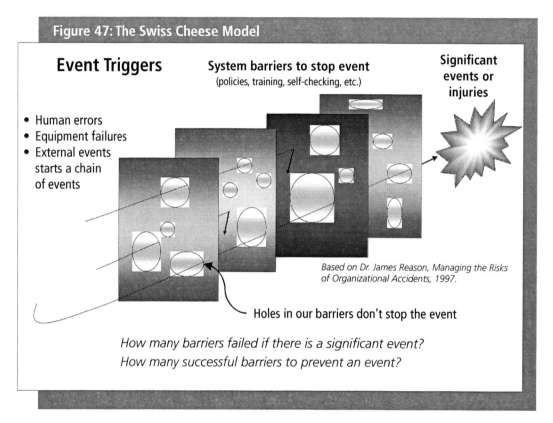

**Figure 47: The Swiss Cheese Model**

**Event Triggers**

**System barriers to stop event**
(policies, training, self-checking, etc.)

**Significant events or injuries**

- Human errors
- Equipment failures
- External events starts a chain of events

*Based on Dr. James Reason, Managing the Risks of Organizational Accidents, 1997.*

Holes in our barriers don't stop the event

*How many barriers failed if there is a significant event?*
*How many successful barriers to prevent an event?*

## The GEMS Model

The second model helps get inside our brain to understand errors. It is called the Generic Error Modeling System, or GEMS for short. It was developed by Jens Rasmussen and James Reason. This model, again simplified, helps us understand three "modes" that we might be in when an error occurs. If we can recognize the mode we are in, it can help us to plan a strategy for preventing errors in that mode.

Does your work fit into any of these types of activities?

- Skill-based activities: Tasks we have so much experience with, we could do them in our sleep

- Rule-based activities: Following rules we have learned and practiced like a recipe or a checklist

- Figuring-it-out activities: Figuring out what to do next without the benefit of rules or experience

## Skill-based errors

Skill-based errors happen when we are performing an activity that we have done many times before. In fact, we may have done it so many times that we are on autopilot and our brain is thinking about other things while our hands are performing the task. Have you ever driven home and pulled into your parking space and not remembered a moment of the trip? You were on autopilot. Your hands were driving the car, but your brain was thinking about the weekend, or a nasty argument you just had, or planning your new house addition—not about driving.

Sometimes when we are on autopilot we forget to do activities—like checking our mirrors before we change lanes. Oops! Other times, when we are on autopilot and our mind is not on the activity at hand, we might do the wrong thing, such as give the meds to the wrong patient as we are carrying on a conversation with our coworkers. Big OOPS!

When are you on autopilot? Think about it. Is it while administering meds? Manipulating IV lines? Replying to "all" when sending e-mails? These are all potential times we can make serious errors.

## Rule-based errors

Many of the activities we do in healthcare are so complex, or we do them so infrequently, that we can't rely on our experience or skill-based behavior to help us know what to do. We need some help. We need instructions, or a cheat sheet, a job aid, a procedure, or a recipe. Really, what we need is a pre-established, prechecked set of "rules" to help us make sure we do things in a correct step-by-step fashion. We need our rules to be like safety fences or guardrails to keep us safe and out of trouble.

So where do we get our rules? Sometimes, when we use the word rules, we think they need to be formal laws or something written down and posted on the bulletin board. Actually, during your life, you have collected quite a collection of rules—both formal and informal. In addition to the formal rules, your rules might include something you studied, or something a professor once told you—and it stuck with you. Maybe something that a classmate or coworker shared with you on the first day of class or work. Maybe something you read on the Internet. These are all collected and stored in your brain, and when a situation comes up, you reach into that 'ol brain, stir it around, and select the rule you think works best. That's what makes us smart: We have a good selection of rules, we know which one to select, and we are not afraid to apply them at the right time.

Can we make a medication error when we are in "rule mode?" Unfortunately, yes, we can. The typical things that go wrong when we are trying to follow rules are:

1.  The rule is bad. The person who was telling us what their rules were didn't know what they were doing, and we picked up bad rules and bad habits. Make sure you get your rules from the right place, and when someone points out that one of your cherished rules may be wrong, listen to them and check it out. We would hate to be using wrong rules.

2.  We choose the wrong rule. We need to not just collect rules but be able to choose the best match for the situation we are in. Our supervisors, coworkers, instructors, proctors, mentors, and others all help us learn which rule best applies in which situation. If you are not sure, ask someone! Don't just guess.

3.  We don't follow the rules. Sometimes, we decide to take a shortcut. It is almost the end of the shift, you are tired, maybe just this one time . . . well, that is a formula for disaster. Remember: The rules are the safety fences to keep us from falling into the open mine shaft. If we ignore the rules, we have a 30% greater chance to make an error than if we follow them (Aspden, et al.)

### Figuring-it-out-based errors

Sometimes we find ourselves in situations where:

- We have no experience with a situation

- We don't have any specific, detailed rules that are applicable

Therefore, we then must rely on our general knowledge to figure out the problem from scratch. When we are trying to figure things out from scratch, we have about a 30% chance of making an error (Aspden, et al.). That's scary! When people nag you about following the rules, remember, they want us to be safe.

If you find that you are in figuring-it-out mode, use the 2:00 a.m. in the dark parking lot rule. "Don't go there alone!" Ask someone, get a consultation, look it up!

So if we want to be dedicated to safe medication and safe pharmacology, what do we do? Don't worry; there are some easy, simple tools to help us reduce medication errors and keep our patients, and ourselves, safe. We will look at these in the next chapter.

## References

Committee on Identifying and Preventing Medication Errors, Aspden, P., Wolcott, J., Bootman, J.L., Cronenwett, L.R. (eds). (2007). *Preventing Medication Errors: Quality Chasm Series*. Washington, D.C.: Institute of Medicine of the National Academies, National Academy of Sciences.

"Statement of Michael L. Langberg, MD." Cedars-Sinai Medical Center. Available at *www.cedars-sinai.edu/pdf/Statement-11-20-07-56336.pdf*. Accessed December 19, 2007.

# Chapter 23

# What can I do to avoid making a medication error?

## Build a culture of safety!

Safety is not something we can add on at the last minute just before our patient leaves the facility. Safety has to be there all the time; it has to be included in everything we do. It has to be an integral and precious part of our culture. In short, we need a culture of safety. So what is "culture?"

Culture is really our shared values and beliefs. If we believe in safe driving, we will wear our seat belts, and we will share that value with everyone who rides in our car. "Buckle up, or the car doesn't move!" is our way of letting people know that our culture of safety will not let us put a passenger at risk.

So what are the shared values and beliefs in healthcare that will keep us from having medication errors? There are six safe behaviors that are expected of all of us to make sure our patients are safe. These are listed below.

## Safe behaviors keep us safe

We expect everyone will:

- Pay attention to details
- Communicate clearly and directly

- Have a questioning attitude

- Perform effective handoffs

- Work together with the team

- Follow the rules

### Pay attention to details

Be careful when you are on autopilot. Are you missing important details because you are distracted? In healthcare, every detail is vital, especially in medication safety. Notice the patient, the arm band, the medication name and dose, the color, the look, the smell, and notice anything that might seem unusual. All those details are important.

**Tip:** Always stop and check what you are doing.

### Communicate clearly and directly

Medication safety requires that we have clear and direct communication. If you don't understand what the doctor ordered, you can not administer it safely. We all talk so much with each other that we sometimes think communication is easy. *Communication takes hard work!* You are expected to communicate clearly and directly and so is the rest of the care team—the doctors, nurses, pharmacists, everyone.

**Tip:** Make sure you are understood and that you understand what others are telling you.

### Have a questioning attitude

What would you do if you saw water on the floor leaking out of the drinking fountain? Would you say, "Oh well, not my problem"? Or would you pick up the phone and call someone? We are all expected to be part of the team in our culture of safety, and this is especially true in preventing medication errors. If you see something that doesn't seem right, such as medications with similar names stored next to each other, or a medication in the wrong drawer in the dispensing equipment, what will you do? Will you say "not my problem," or will you tell someone and make sure it gets corrected?

**Tip:** If something doesn't seem right, it probably isn't. Ask the question. If there wasn't a problem, you learned something. If there was a problem, you may have saved a life!

### Perform effective handoffs

Every day, we hand off many pieces of information about our patients and their medications. Each of these handoffs must be performed completely and effectively.

In the Super Bowl, one fumble can change the entire outcome of the game. The same is true in healthcare; one dropped handoff can forever change the future for a patient.

 **Tip:** Make sure that every time responsibility for a patient or an action changes hands, you have a complete picture of all the medications and possible issues related to your patient. Remember: NO dropped balls!

### Work together with the team

We are much stronger together than if we all work independently. We need people on our team who are willing to provide a peer check when our mind has turned to marshmallow.

We also need our "safety buddies." If you have tried to maintain an exercise or diet program, you know how much easier it is if you work with others. Preventing medication errors is no different.

 **Tip:** Work with your "medication safety buddies," talk about issues, check each other, encourage each other to be focused completely on safety every day. Remember: Our culture of safety is driven by our shared values and beliefs. Share yours! Be a safety advocate!

### Follow the rules

Our rules about medication administration have been designed as the safety fences and guardrails to keep our patients and each of us safe. They can't work if we don't follow the rules. Every time you take a shortcut or decide to not follow a rule, you are increasing your error rate from about 1% to about 30% (Aspden, et al.)

 **Tip:** Not following the rules is like walking a tightrope without a net. Don't do it!

## Simple tools to help prevent medication errors

We all want to meet these six expectations for safe behaviors. To make it easier, there are some simple tools for you to remember. Each of these takes just a few seconds and will make you a top scholar—and performer—in medication safety.

---

### Behavior expectation

| | |
|---|---|
| Pay attention to details | STAR |
| Communicate clearly | SBAR, 3-way repeat back, phonetic and numeric clarifications |
| Have a questioning attitude | Stop and ask |
| Perform effective handoffs | What, why, warnings |
| Work together with the team | Peer checking, peer coaching, escalate your concerns |
| Follow the rules | |

---

## Be a STAR

STAR is a simple way to remember to self-check our activities. It is perfect for keeping us from being on autopilot and forgetting to check a detail. STAR stands for Stop, Think, Act, and Review and takes just a second to do:

- STOP: Pause for 1–2 seconds to focus on what you're about to do.

- THINK: Think about what you're about to do; is it the right thing?

- ACT: Concentrate and perform the task.

- REVIEW: Check to see if the task was done right.

Here are a couple examples:

- When you leave your house or apartment, do you do the "Badge, Beeper and Key Dance?" You know the one. You stop at the front door (STOP), you pat all your pockets (THINK), you close the door (ACT), you bounce your keys in your hand (REVIEW), and then go to work.

See, you already know how to do STAR; do it for your patients anytime there are details that need to be self-checked.

- Clinically speaking, let's use starting or modifying an IV or central line. As soon as you touch the line, STOP. Then, look to verify where it came from and where it is going (THINK). Then do what needs to be done (ACT). Finally, make sure it is running correctly (REVIEW).

If you made this a habit and did this every time, you would be a safety STAR!

## Raise the communication bar with SBAR

SBAR is a method to remind us not to leave out important things when communicating about a problem. It also keeps us on track and from rambling during an important communication. Use it when you call a physician about a medication problem at 2:00 a.m., and they will appreciate that you raised the bar with SBAR.

When you need to communicate about a problem or issue that needs resolution, use SBAR:

- <u>Situation:</u> Who you're calling about, the immediate problem, current vital signs, your concerns.

- <u>Background:</u> Review of pertinent information: procedures, mental status, skin condition, oxygenation.

- <u>Assessment:</u> Your view of the situation: "I think the problem is . . ." or "I'm not sure what the problem is." (Also point out the urgency of action: "The patient is deteriorating rapidly; we need to do something. . .")

- <u>Recommendation:</u> Your recommendation or request.

## Three parts is a charm: Use three-part repeat back communication

When a physician gives you a verbal order (yikes!) or wants a change in a patient's medications, we had better make sure we heard exactly what they asked for. Unfortunately, with noise, confusion, people talking to four people at once, and lots of different accents, sometimes we might not hear things correctly. That's why we should all use three-part repeat back communication.

You tell me, I repeat it back to you, and then you confirm. Simple but effective! Here's how it works:

1. **Sender initiates** communication using receiver's name. Sender provides a request or information to receiver in a clear and concise format.

2. **Receiver acknowledges** receipt by a repeat back of the request or information.

3. **Sender acknowledges** the accuracy of the repeat back, saying, "That's correct." If not correct, repeat the communication.

## Taking it to a higher level of safety

Sometimes you see things that are not safe and want to protect your patient or coworker from making a mistake. But that is not easy, especially if the person who is about to do something unsafe is a physician and you are in your first year. But you can't just close your eyes and hope they will go away! You need to take action.

Don't just dive in; use a strategy to escalate your concern:

- Start easy with a gentle nudge; ask a question. Maybe the person will see the error and fix it.

- If that doesn't work, request them to change their behavior for the sake of the patient. It can help if you have a suggestion for a safer alternative handy that you can share with them.

- If that still doesn't work, express your concern and then get your chain of command involved.

It is not always easy, but if there is a real problem, your patient will thank you, and you will know that you took it to a higher level of safety!

## Oh no! It just happened to me!

So, what if a medication error occurs? Here's what to do:

- Assist the patient.

- Get your team involved: Tell someone so they can help you help the patient, and tell your supervisor—Always!

- Chart it. Yes, you always chart medication errors—Always!

- Report it. Fill in the medication error or occurrence report utilized by your hospital.

- Analyze it. The quality, performance or risk departments will analyze the problem to see what can be changed to prevent it from happening again. They will also look at trends to see if they are seeing more of these kinds of errors.

- Prevent it. The underlying problem needs to be fixed. If you have a suggestion, talk to your supervisor or the performance improvement department. Fix it so you and your team don't have to worry about it in the future.

**Don't forget:** If you don't report it, it can't be fixed.

## References

Committee on Identifying and Preventing Medication Errors, Aspden, P., Wolcott, J., Bootman, J.L., Cronenwett, L.R. (eds). (2007). *Preventing Medication Errors: Quality Chasm Series*. Washington, D.C.: Institute of Medicine of the National Academies, National Academy of Sciences.

# Chapter 24

# So now what?
# I'm just supposed
# to know all this?

We're in for another brief lesson, but only because you already know the answers. Of course, that may or may not be readily apparent. We've covered a ton of information in our time together: Do you recall how we did it? Though not explicitly stated, all of our classes initially focused on learning the big picture. We took our first swipe at particular topics with a broad brush to paint the background and subsequently added the nuanced detail.

## Appropriate expectations

Remember, you don't have to know everything there is to know! Your brain is not able to hold all of the information about every available medication. Some appropriate expectations include:

- Understanding basic pharmacokinetic concepts

- Knowing the broad categories of medications, and their uses, limitations, and potential adverse effects

- Knowing the essential information about each particular drug prior to administration: patient's dose, usual dose, medication indications for this patient, potential contraindications for this patient, and potential adverse effects

You will find that your clinical practice will determine the cluster of medications with which you are most familiar. You will also come to realize that, with practice, it becomes easier to learn the required information about new and unfamiliar drugs.

## Scan your brain . . . you know more than you think!

Do you remember this comment from our first lesson, "First, there is the language. By now, you have perused your pharmacology text. You've heard of pharmacokinetics, loop diuretics, mood stabilizing agents, beta 2 adrenergic antagonists, etc." There are some bemused expressions of recognition out there—yes!—there isn't a word in that sentence you don't recognize and know. Moreover, those words evoked all sorts of connections:

- Pharmacokinetics stimulated memories of absorption, distribution, metabolism, and excretion.

- Loop diuretics made you think of thiazide diuretics, potassium wasting, dehydration, hypotension, and all sorts of related topics.

- Beta 2 adrenergics: 1 heart beta 1, 2 lungs beta 2, alpha 1, alpha 2, adrenergic, cholinergic . . . it all really does come back!

 **Don't forget:** You can learn anything by chunking it into bite-size pieces and repetition. And once you get the information into long-term memory, it will stay despite only intermittent use!

 **Tip:** Keep all of your newly acquired knowledge through regular use.

 **Tip:** Now would be the ideal time to begin reading professional journals (we'll touch more on these in a bit) to solidify what you know and give what you know a contextual framework to enhance processing and retention. For example, reading a graphic case history of the experience of a person afflicted with heart failure will greatly aid your recall.

## Staying sharp in the pharmacological future

You may not know everything about pharmacology. (In fact, it's a safe bet that you probably will never know all there is to know.) But, by knowing where to turn to get information, you'll be set up for a successful nursing career filled with safe practice. Let's take a quick pharmacological tour:

- Pharmacists: This other group of professionals belonging to our health-care provider team are outstanding and willing information sources. Pharmacists are superbly prepared to answer our questions about medication indications, contraindications, adverse effects, and potential interactions. If you are a hospital-based nurse, this resource is just a phone call or page away.

- Online sources: I put the keywords "drug information" in the Google search window and got 38,300,000 hits in 0.11 seconds. How can you choose a reliable and current source? There are some general rules of thumb (Google that phrase and get 4,450,000 hits!). First, consider the source: governmental or academic sources are good places to begin. Using our "drug information" example, the first hit was MedlinePlus at *www.nlm.nih.gov/medlineplus/druginformation.html*. This is a site operated by the United States Library of Medicine and the National Institutes of Health—fairly reliable!

- Don't forget databases: Any college library most certainly has subscriptions to journal databases such as Medline, PubMed, First Search, and Scopus. These are excellent sources of information that can lead you to individual clinical journals. Even if you have graduated, many colleges and universities who receive public funding provide limited access to people in the communities they serve.

- Clinical journals: One enduring mark of the true professional is the diligent reading of professional information. Traditionally, this has been in the form of print publications, but there are a growing number of online journals that publish evidence-based (proven by research) information.

- PDA subscriptions: Another electronic resource is the subscription database that can be downloaded on your PDA or pocket computer. The subscriber pays an annual fee for which he or she receives updates to a base program. Most published comprehensive nursing drug guides offer PDA resources, and there are others, such as Epocrates, geared more toward the provider who prescribes medications.

- Professional associations: As you graduate and become licensed (or perhaps you already have), don't forget to consider joining a professional organization. Organizations give you the opportunity to learn from peers and experienced mentors in your chosen specialty and to give expression to your informed opinion as a healthcare provider. As a profession, nursing has many from which to choose. Here are a few examples:

- Academy of Medical-Surgical Nurses

- Academy of Neonatal Nursing

- Air & Surface Transport Nurses Association

- Alliance for Psychosocial Nursing

- American Academy of Ambulatory Care Nursing

- American Academy of Nurse Practitioners

- American Academy of Nursing

- American Assembly for Men in Nursing

- American Assisted Living Nurses Association

- American Association for the History of Nursing

- American Association of Colleges of Nursing

- American Association of Critical Care Nurses

- American Association of Heart Failure Nurses

- American Association of Legal Nurse Consultants

- American Association of Managed Care Nurses

- American Association of Neuroscience Nurses

- American Association of Nurse Anesthetists

- American Association of Nurse Attorneys

Let's take a short break before the final exam . . .

# References

"Nursing Organization Links." NP Central. Available at *www.nurse.org/orgs.shtml*. Accessed December 17, 2007.

# Chapter 25

# Sound the trumpets! It's time for the final exam!

You are there! You hung on until the end of our class. Well done! This is the payoff. Not only do you now know how to study pharmacology, but the lessons and strategies you used will absolutely guide you toward scintillating success when you take the NCLEX-RN®. So in this final lesson, we are going to look at that exam and then analyze a few practice problems of our own. Let's sprint to the finish!

## Some NCLEX-RN® help, please

Each state in the United States has a board of nursing. Often the members are appointed by the governor and include notable nurses from varied specialties, education levels, and professional backgrounds. Each board may also include members representing other perspectives: nurse assistants, insurance providers, lawyers, and consumers, for example. Within each state, the board of nursing sets standards for licensure, education, and clinical practice. The boards collaborate to moderate the state-to-state differences and to construct the licensure exam used in all states.

### How the test is constructed

**Click:** Download the free NCLEX-RN® Examination Test Plan for the National Council Licensure Examination for Registered Nurses at *https://ncsbn.org/RN_Test_Plan_2007_Web.pdf*. It's always a good idea to go to the source for basic information. The document also gives you some clues as to the distribution of the questions. For example, the test taker can expect 8%–14% of the questions to deal with safety or infection control and 13%–19% to ask about pharmacologic interventions.

This kind of content gives us an idea of the scope and balance of the examination. This test plan also tells us that the test is constructed for each candidate using computerized adaptive testing. The candidate must answer a minimum of 75 questions and may answer up to 265. (Each test also includes 15 pretest questions that are being gauged for future examinations.) The range exists because the exam is assembled interactively as the test progresses during the six-hour period. The time you spend is not an indicator of how well or poorly you perform. It is only a measure of the time the computer needed to determine your competency—some will take the full six hours, others will be shorter. Questions are selected that match your ability (usually starting off with medium difficulty, then harder or easier), your competence is assessed by the computer, and the exam continues until a pass or fail decision is made.

## Types of questions
The examination includes

- Multiple-choice questions that typically ask you to choose the best option: There is one correct choice and three that may partially aid the patient situation in the question root.

- Multiple-response questions: These are similar to multiple-choice questions, but one or more choices may be correct.

- Hot-spot questions: The computer asks you, for example, to identify the correct place on the patient image to check for myxedema due to hypothyroidism. It directs you to move the cursor there and click.

- Fill in the blanks: These are used when the exam asks you to calculate drug dosages based on body weight.

- Chart/exhibit questions: These efficiently mimic searching in a patient's chart to find information needed to solve a particular issue

- Drag and drop/ordered-response questions: These ask you to arrange data in a particular order (Billings).

## How to study for the test
Do practice questions, do practice questions, and do practice questions!
If you go through 3,000–5,000 NCLEX-style questions, you'll increase your

chances of success. What really increases your chances is NOT (sorry for shouting) attempting to learn all the nursing material you should have learned in the prior two to four years (depending on your college) in the last two weeks before your NCLEX! If you spend your entire nursing school career cramming important new information in preparation for each test, you are operating just like your Internet browser: repetitively filling and deleting temporary files. This is not a good situation.

Remember and consciously implement the knowledge and strategies you gained in our learning hygiene lessons (see Chapter 3) to promote long-term retention of important information.

 **Tip:** Here are a few other tips:

- Study regularly over a period of months

- Begin studying even before you finish your nursing education

- Take advantage of any examination preparation resources offered by your college

- Consider purchasing a review text with a CD-ROM that simulates actual testing; get recommendations or suggestions from your nursing faculty

## Pencils ready, eyes forward . . .

Let's look at some typical questions:

### The test

1. Your post-myocardial infarction (heart attack) client has gained four pounds in the past two days, has edema in his bilateral lower extremities, and has difficulty in breathing. You can expect the physician to order

   a. Nitroglycerin to reduce cardiac afterload.
   b. Furosemide to promote high-volume diuresis.
   c. Spironolactone to stimulate a safe low-volume diuresis.
   d. The client to begin a low-sodium diet.

2.  Your patient is experiencing postoperative pain following her gallbladder removal and has received intermittent intravenous injections of hydromorphone. The priority question for the nurse to ask is:

    a.  When was your last bowel movement?
    b.  Is there any history of drug addiction in your family?
    c.  Have you noticed any sleepiness after the injections?
    d.  How would you rate your pain relief after the injection?

3.  Your patient is on a heparin drip. A 250 mL bag of D5W contains 25,000 units of heparin. Your patient needs to receive 2000 units per hour. How many mL/hour should you run the IV at? _____

4.  The patient with emphysema is taking large doses of prednisone to reduce inflammation and ease respiratory distress. What priority instruction should the nurse give?

    a.  Weigh yourself daily to monitor weight gain related to increased fat deposition.
    b.  Monitor your blood sugars since glucocorticoids promote hyperglycemia.
    c.  You can expect to have periods of sudden anger due to the effect of the medication on the hypothalamus.
    d.  Prednisone is not safe for long-term use. Your physician will prescribe a safer alternative after the acute phase of your illness.

5.  The nurse's priority education intervention for a person taking warfarin following the insertion of an artificial heart valve is:

    a.  Eat a diet rich in vitamin K to reduce risk of hemorrhage.
    b.  Avoid strenuous activity to avoid bleeding in joints.
    c.  Have blood tests drawn as directed to monitor medication effect.
    d.  Consider taking 1 aspirin twice daily to enhance the anticoagulant effect.

## The answers

1. Your post-myocardial infarction (heart attack) client has gained four pounds in the past two days, has edema in his bilateral lower extremities, and has difficulty in breathing. You can expect the physician to order

   a. Nitroglycerin to reduce cardiac afterload. *(Incorrect)*
   b. **Furosemide to promote high-volume diuresis. *(Correct)***
   c. Spironolactone to stimulate a safe low-volume diuresis. *(Doesn't promote enough fluid loss)*
   d. The client to begin a low-sodium diet. *(Important in the long term but won't ease symptoms now)*

2. Your patient is experiencing postoperative pain following her gallbladder removal and has received intermittent intravenous injections of hydromorphone. The priority question for the nurse to ask is:

   a. When was your last bowel movement? *(All opioids cause constipation, but not the most important issue in this situation)*
   b. Is there any history of drug addiction in your family? *(Opioid use can lead to psychological dependence in some people, but this question is unimportant)*
   c. Have you noticed any sleepiness after the injections? *(An expected finding)*
   d. **How would you rate your pain relief after the injection? *(Correct; we want to know if the dose is effective)***

3. Your patient is on a heparin drip. A 250 mL bag of D5W contains 25,000 units of heparin. Your patient needs to receive 2000 units per hour. How many mL/hour should you run the IV at? *20 mL/hr*

4. The patient with emphysema is taking large doses of prednisone to reduce inflammation and ease respiratory distress. What priority instruction should the nurse give?

   a. Weigh yourself daily to monitor weight gain related to increased fat deposition. *(Incorrect)*
   b. **Monitor your blood sugars since glucocorticoids promote hyperglycemia. *(Correct)***
   c. You can expect to have periods of sudden anger due to the effect of the medication on the hypothalamus. *(Not true)*
   d. Prednisone is not safe for long-term use. Your physician will prescribe a safer alternative after the acute phase of your illness. *(Long-term use always has adverse effects, but there may not be other options)*

5. The nurse's priority education intervention for a person taking warfarin following the insertion of an artificial heart valve is:

    a. Eat a diet rich in vitamin K to reduce risk of hemorrhage. *(Vitamin K is the antidote and works against the therapeutic effect—patients should be instructed to eat a consistent amount of vitamin K-containing foods to avoid swings in the effectiveness of the warfarin)*

    b. Avoid strenuous activity to avoid bleeding in joints. *(Not true)*

    c. **Have blood tests drawn as directed to monitor medication effect.** *(Correct)*

    d. Consider taking 1 aspirin twice daily to enhance the anticoagulant effect. *(NSAID use increases risk of hemorrhage)*

## Some closing thoughts

Michael Ende wrote a fantasy novel in 1979 called "The Neverending Story." And, of course, you're probably all familiar with the movie of that name. Pharmacology is a lot like that—no, not a tale of dragons and ivory towers. The analogy is that our study never ends. The subject is fascinating for us and crucial for our patients.

We need to keep learning and sharing what we know with our patients, because the more we both know, the better the outcome will be for our clients—and ourselves.

## References

Billings, D. (2008) *NCLEX-RN* 9th ed. Philadelphia: Lippincott Williams & Wilkins.

"NCLEX-RN Examination: Test Plan for the National Counsel Licensure Examination for Registered Nurses." National Council of State Boards of Nursing. Available at *https://ncsbn.org/RN_Test_Plan_2007_Web.pdf*. Accessed December 18, 2007.

# Who said nursing can't be fun?

We're the leading "dot calm" resource
when you're feeling stressed.

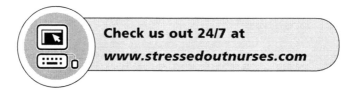

**Check us out 24/7 at**
***www.stressedoutnurses.com***

**What will you find there? Along with this
colorful character, you'll see:**

- ✔ **Contests**
- ✔ **Fun, witty articles that will help
  relieve your stress**
- ✔ **Resources to help you on your
  journey as a nurse**
- ✔ **Much, much more**

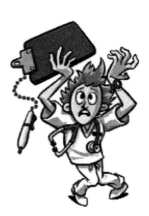

So, what are you waiting for?

**Get clicking and kiss your stress goodbye!**